D1261953

Families of Children With Developmental Disabilities

Families of Children With Developmental Disabilities

Understanding Stress and Opportunities for Growth

David W. Carroll

American Psychological Association · Washington, DC

BH

Published by
American Psychological Association
750 First Street, NE
Washington, DC 20002
www.apa.org

To order
APA Order Department
P.O. Box 92984
Washington, DC 20090-2984
Tel: (800) 374-2721; Direct: (202) 336-5510
Fax: (202) 336-5502; TDD/TTY: (202) 336-6123
Online: www.apa.org/pubs/books
E-mail: order@apa.org

In the U.K., Europe, Africa, and the Middle East, copies may be ordered from
American Psychological Association
3 Henrietta Street
Covent Garden, London
WC2E 8LU England

Typeset in Goudy by Circle Graphics, Inc., Columbia, MD

Printer: Maple Press, York, PA
Cover Designer: Mercury Publishing Services, Rockville, MD

The opinions and statements published are the responsibility of the authors, and such opinions and statements do not necessarily represent the policies of the American Psychological Association.

Library of Congress Cataloging-in-Publication Data

Carroll, David W., 1950-
  Families of children with developmental disabilities : understanding stress and opportunities for growth / David W. Carroll.
      pages cm
  Includes bibliographical references and index.
  ISBN 978-1-4338-1329-0 — ISBN 1-4338-1329-7 1. Parents of children with disabilities—Services for. 2. Children with disabilities—Family relationships. 3. Family social work.
  I. Title.
  HQ759.913.C37 2013
  362.4'043—dc23
                         2012051343

British Library Cataloguing-in-Publication Data

A CIP record is available from the British Library.

Printed in the United States of America
First Edition

http://dx.doi.org/10.1037/14192-000

12/9/13

In memory of Michael Adam Carroll

CONTENTS

PREFACE

This volume reflects the culmination of my professional and personal journeys. I became the father of a child with cerebral palsy shortly after beginning a faculty appointment at the University of Wisconsin–Superior in 1978 and spent the next 22 years balancing my professorial responsibilities with those of the father of a child with serious medical needs. I consulted physicians, worked with physical and occupational therapists, and attended meetings with educators. Along the way, I learned a fair amount about the legal and cultural aspects of disability and reflected on how my son's disabilities pervaded virtually every aspect of my life. Parenting a child with a developmental disability influences a person emotionally, physically, socially, and financially.

Over the years, I gave thought to writing about our family's experiences and looked at competing books on the market. As it turned out, the book I had planned to write had already been written many times. Dozens if not hundreds of books have been written by parents of children with various disabilities. Our family's experience, although unique in many of the details, was fundamentally similar to those of families of children with different disabilities and from different socioeconomic backgrounds. These parents shared the challenges of raising a child with a disability along with the joys such a child can bring. I emerged from my reading with the conviction that these parents' stories deserve a place in a full account of the family experience with disability.

In addition, during 34 years of teaching classes in child development, I regularly discussed various aspects of family life, including how parents influence child behavior (and vice versa), how siblings interact, and the role of the extended family. Among the topics of these discussions was the diversity of family configurations, such as single-parent families and families with various racial and ethnic backgrounds. However, I found that few of the textbooks made more than a cursory mention of families of children with developmental disabilities. Over the years, I delved into the research on families touched by disability to supplement my lectures in this area.

As I examined the research more fully, I realized that the field had a significant need for integration. Although research has explored particular aspects of families of children with developmental disabilities, I could not find a book that pulled the research together into a coherent whole, summarizing the current consensus and identifying areas worthy of additional study. Out of this realization came the decision to write this volume.

The effect of a child with a developmental disability on the family has drawn a tremendous amount of interest from scholars. The sheer amount of research in just the past decade is staggering. Of the over 550 research articles and books cited in this volume, more than 400 have been published since 2000 and 75 since 2010. The literature has matured to the point that it is now possible to present conclusions on a number of important issues, such as the relationship between parental stress and depressive symptoms or the effect of training in behavioral management skills on the psychological well-being of parents. I believe these are important conclusions, ones that should drive both practice and policy.

My review of the literature identified areas in which additional research is sorely needed. For example, research on the similarities and differences between various disabilities is fragmentary, as is scholarship on how child disabilities affect grandparents. I have emphasized the value of particular research approaches that have been fruitful for psychology on the whole but that have been underutilized in the study of families of children with disabilities. For one, the narrative approach has energized the study of personality but has not been applied systematically to stories written by parents of children with developmental disabilities. For another, some of the research reported in this volume attests to the positive outcomes spurred by a child's disability; such reports are obviously relevant to the field of positive psychology, but little has been done to integrate these areas of scholarship.

The issues of concern to families of children with disabilities have elicited interest from a wide variety of disciplines, including psychology, pediatrics, nursing, special education, and sociology. Although the interest of scholars from different fields has had synergistic effects on the study of disabilities, it also presents a challenge for scholars. Different disciplines employ different methodologies, ranging from randomized controlled studies to meta-analyses of treatment effects to qualitative research studies that extract themes from interview data. There are differences as well in the time frame employed by researchers. For example, most of the studies of how parents react to the placement of an infant in a newborn intensive care unit were organized by nursing researchers to examine immediate effects. Psychologists interested in the prevalence of posttraumatic symptoms in parents are more likely to examine longer-term consequences. I have tried to emphasize that different questions demand different approaches and to integrate these diverse approaches into a coherent story, albeit one with some missing details.

Although much research has examined how families respond to the challenges of a child with a developmental disability, no single volume pulls all of the research together. I anticipate that this volume will be useful to developmental psychologists interested in family dynamics, particularly those interested in how the stresses associated with children with developmental disabilities influence family interactions. The volume should also be of value to clinical psychologists and other mental health professionals who provide services to families touched by disability. The volume is organized developmentally. It begins with the initial reactions of parents to a child with an unexpected health condition, then analyzes the family as a system of interconnected members adapting to a child with developmental issues, and finally discusses how family dynamics shift when an individual with a disability approaches adulthood. I also expect that clinical psychologists will find much of value here. The experience of parenting a child with a disability is undeniably stressful, and some parents may benefit from professional help. On the other hand, parents often find meaning and benefit in their lives with children with disabilities. I believe that the characterization of the mix of emotions found here will be useful for clinicians who treat families of children with disabilities.

It is a poorly kept secret that a book is the result of the efforts of many people other than the author. I am pleased to acknowledge the assistance of the two anonymous reviewers who provided detailed and highly useful critiques of earlier drafts and drew my attention both to points that needed to be sharpened and issues that deserved fuller consideration. In addition, the staff at APA Books was superb. Maureen Adams showed confidence in the project long before it was deserved. Tyler Aune and Liz Brace expertly guided the transition from rough draft to finished volume. I thank all of these individuals for the improvement of the manuscript. Of course, any remaining errors are my responsibility. Finally, I want to thank my wife, Deb, for her understanding and support during the writing of this volume.

Families of Children With Developmental Disabilities

1

INTRODUCTION

Certainly I never in my wildest dreams had planned for any of the
experiences that we've had since having a child with a disability. . . . It
has changed absolutely every waking moment of our lives. (G. A. King,
Zwaigenbaum, et al., 2006, p. 358)

No one expects to have a child with a developmental disability. Future
parents, whether or not they are fully aware of it, develop expectations for
their unborn children. Most wonder about the child's gender, and many think
about whether the child will look or act like the parents or other relatives.
However, few parents-to-be think seriously about the prospect of raising a
child with a significant medical problem. Perhaps the closest most parents
get to that thought is the often-expressed statement, "I just want the baby to
be healthy."

Parents of children with developmental disabilities quickly encounter many challenges posed by their child's disability as well as the societal
response to people with disabilities. The child may have significant health
care needs and require many medical appointments that interfere with parents' work and present financial hardships. Many children with disabilities
have behavioral issues that can be emotionally draining for the parents and

http://dx.doi.org/10.1037/14192-001
Families of Children With Developmental Disabilities: Understanding Stress and Opportunities for Growth,
by D. W. Carroll

the entire family. When children with disabilities enter the school system, parents often find that educators do not share their values concerning how to educate their children. Society as a whole conveys certain attitudes toward individuals with disabilities that parents inevitably experience. These challenges leave many parents tired and frustrated.

In addition to these daily challenges, parents of children with disabilities also must confront their own expectations for their children (Russell, 2003). Parents need to explicitly identify and reassess their dreams for their children and their lives and reorient themselves and their families toward a reality they scarcely could have anticipated. They must adapt to their present circumstances and prepare for an uncertain future.

This volume addresses how families make these adaptations. These issues have been studied in detail in recent years, and a comprehensive and current account of the literature is provided, covering research from psychology and related fields. Parents of children with disabilities experience a mixture of emotions not easily understood by people who have not had similar experiences. The volume provides guidance on the issues that parents, siblings, and grandparents consider most important and need professional assistance to address. The final chapter summarizes what is currently known as well as areas that would benefit from further research.

This chapter begins by considering the construct of developmental disabilities and how it has evolved over time. Then we consider four theoretical perspectives that can provide some guidance on issues related to families of children with disabilities and some methodological issues in this area of study. The chapter closes with an overview of the following chapters and the main themes of the book.

THE CONSTRUCT OF DEVELOPMENTAL DISABILITIES

The concept of developmental disabilities is at once a scientific, cultural, legal, and personal construct. It is defined in different ways for different purposes in each of these domains. For some, the definition enables individuals and their families to secure educational and social services. For others, the term is defined precisely enough to allow researchers to study characteristics of individuals and their families. For still others, the definition is a construct that enables scholars to examine cultural attitudes toward certain groups of people.

As a working definition, we may state that developmental disabilities are disabilities that have an early onset and include some degree of developmental delay. As the term is ordinarily used, it includes a number of conditions such as Down syndrome, autism spectrum disorder, cerebral palsy, fragile X syndrome, attention-deficit/hyperactivity disorder, and neural tube defects (such as spina bifida). It also includes conditions that are not well understood, such as pervasive developmental disorder, but that nonetheless entail developmental delay. In contrast, physical conditions without developmental delays (e.g., diabetes, cancer), mental disorders (e.g., bipolar disorder), and acquired disabilities (e.g., traumatic brain injury from an accident) are typically excluded, although it is sometimes instructive to contrast family responses to developmental disabilities with their responses to these other conditions.

Although a working definition of developmental disabilities is helpful, it is counterproductive to draw the lines too sharply. The construct of developmental disabilities has evolved, and thus some or even many of the conditions currently viewed as developmental disabilities are likely to be reexamined in ways that are difficult to predict in the years and decades to come. To gain some perspective, we need to consider the evolution of the construct.

Historical Constructions of Disabilities

Braddock and Parish (2001) provided an overview of historical views and treatment of individuals with disabilities from classical antiquity to the 20th century. They noted that that the ancient Greeks are now widely believed to have practiced infanticide of the disabled, sometimes for economic reasons when there were too many children to support. Garland (2010) observed that since the Greeks believed that the birth of a healthy child was the result of goodwill from the gods, it followed that a deformed child was seen as a consequence of their anger. Therefore, killing the young by exposure was a means of mollifying the gods. However, these practices were not universal: In Sparta, the law required the abandonment of deformed and sickly infants, but Athenians were apparently permitted to raise such children.

During the Middle Ages, many disabilities were believed to be caused by demons, with consequent exorcism (Braddock & Parish, 2001). Nonetheless, more sympathetic views of the disabled coexisted. Neugebauer (1978) reported that state responsibility for care of the disabled grew during this period. Neugebauer reviewed court records in England from the late 13th century to the 1640s and found that documents distinguished between individuals with subnormal intelligence at birth (referred to as *natural fools* or *idiots*) and those who developed their conditions postnatally. The king took custody of the land of the natural fools and arranged for them to receive necessary care. Moreover, the kingdom developed procedures, such as tests of memory and reading, to evaluate the mental status of individuals alleged to be subnormal.

By the late 17th century, more attention was paid to the distinction between intellectual disability and mental illness (see Goodey, 2001). Although English property law distinguished between the two conditions in the 13th century, there was a financial incentive for the state to confuse them, since the kingdom took custody of the property of individuals with subnormal intelligence but not mental illness. By 1690, John Locke provided an influential distinction between idiots and *mad men*. Locke suggested that idiots were distinguished from normal men in their inability to form abstract ideas. In contrast, mad men had no shortage of ideas, but their ideas were formed wrongly (Braddock & Parish, 2001).

Although individuals with intellectual impairments were recognized and received support from late medieval institutions, little treatment was provided for such individuals at this point (Stainton, 2001). No hospitals were established specifically for the intellectually impaired, and little evidence indicates that intellectual impairment was regarded as a psychological or medical problem. Treatment programs for the intellectually disabled emerged by the early 1800s. The first systematic and documented treatment program, to treat the feral child Victor, was established by the physician Jean-Marc Itard in France in 1800 (Lane, 1976). Itard developed methods to teach language to Victor but ultimately abandoned the enterprise (and Victor) after a number of years of disappointing results. In the mid-19th century in the United States, Dorothea Dix advocated treatment for individuals with intellectual disabilities and mental illness. However, enthusiasm for rehabilitation waned by the end of the century. The earliest methods were not proven to be successful; moreover, by the late 1800s the United States had become a more industrial nation, and individuals with intellectual disabilities did not fit well into the workplace.

In 1905, the French scholars Alfred Binet and Théodore Simon created the first intelligence tests. They were designed to identify children who were likely to perform at grade level in the public school system and were administered individually. The psychologist Henry Goddard, who worked at the Vineland School for the Feeble-Minded in New Jersey, convinced American physicians to use Binet and Simon's tests to classify degrees of mental deficiency (Zenderland, 1998). An idiot was defined as an individual with a mental age of 3 or less on Binet and Simon's intelligence scale, and an *imbecile* was a person with a mental age between 3 and 7. Goddard coined the term *moron* to refer to higher-functioning persons with mental ages between 8 and 12. Although such terms make modern eyes wince, they were originally intended as descriptive terms to facilitate diagnosis and guide treatment. As these words took on negative connotations, they were replaced with other terms, such as *mental retardation*, then *developmentally delayed*, and more recently, *intellectual disability* (see Harris, 2010).

The eugenics movement also gained momentum in the early 20th century. In 1869, Francis Galton, a cousin of Charles Darwin, had suggested that intelligence was hereditary and encouraged more intelligent individuals to mate with one another in order to lead to more favorable outcomes for future generations. Galton coined the term *eugenics* from a Greek root meaning good in birth or wellborn (Zenderland, 1998) to refer to the process by which society controls the processes of human heredity for its benefit. By the early 1900s, eugenics enthusiasts argued that since feeble-mindedness was associated with a variety of social ills, efforts to control the reproduction of the feeble-minded were necessary. In 1912, Goddard published a study of a family he called the Kallikaks in which antisocial behavior such as criminal behavior and drug abuse were thought to be passed on from one generation to the next. Such apparently scientific evidence stoked fears that individuals with intellectual disabilities were a danger to society. As a consequence, in the first few decades of the 20th century, many eugenics advocates became enthusiastic not only for positive eugenic methods (i.e., encouraging intellectually superior individuals to find similar mates) but also for negative eugenics methods, including segregation and even sterilization of those suspected to be mentally inferior. The eugenics movement reached its peak in 1927 when the United States Supreme Court ruled that a state could sterilize individuals with intellectual disabilities. Although it is difficult to establish reliable estimates, perhaps as many as 50,000 sterilizations occurred in the United States between 1907 and the repeal of the sterilization laws in the 1970s and 1980s (Lombardo, 2008).

Three Models of Disabilities

One way to summarize the historical evolution of ideas about disability is by reference to the three models of disabilities discussed by Olkin (2002). The moral model holds that disability is a defect caused by a moral lapse or sin or is a test of one's faith. Although it is no longer common to ascribe disabilities to demons, traces of the moral model remain in present-day discourse about disabilities. When individuals suggest that parents were chosen for the burden of caring for a child with a disability for a reason, they are acknowledging divine guidance.

The medical model regards disabilities as physical defects that can be ameliorated by medical treatment. These conditions require diagnosis by medical experts who recommend the appropriate rehabilitation or medical treatment. Although the medical model reduces the sense of shame associated with moral failure, it encourages individuals with disabilities to become dependent on medical professionals for the prescription of medications, equipment, and treatments.

The social model views disability as a social construct and distinguishes between impairment and disability (Braddock & Parish, 2001; Harris, 2010). An impairment is an underlying condition, such as a brain injury, deafness, or low intelligence, that limits an individual's ability to adapt to life. In contrast, disability is defined socially. It refers to how individuals with impairments are regarded in society. For example, poor vision is an impairment that can be corrected by eyeglasses and other environmental supports such as improved lighting. Similarly, a society that does not provide curb cuts for wheelchairs may turn the impairment of paralysis into a disability. Thus, the construct of developmental disabilities does not refer to an individual but rather to an individual's relationship with the larger society.

The social model has been advanced by disability rights groups who have pressed legislatures and the courts to safeguard civil rights for individuals with disabilities (some of the efforts related to education are discussed in Chapter 6). Despite tensions between the medical and social models, each view has contributed to the trend of deinstitutionalizing individuals with disabilities. Disability rights activists have argued for greater inclusion of individuals with disabilities in society, whereas advocates of the medical model believe that proper medical treatment and rehabilitation may enable individuals with disabilities to live a more normal life. Ultimately, these forces have led more children and young adults with developmental disabilities to live in their family homes rather than in institutions. This development, in turn, has increased attention to the challenges parents face in caring for family members with disabilities.

All three models are still relevant to the experience of families of children with developmental disabilities. From a professional vantage point, the medical and social models coexist, albeit somewhat uneasily. Although professionals do not espouse the moral model, elements of moral judgments are evident in how members of society sometimes react to parents of children with disabilities. For example, children with autism often display behaviors that do not fit societal norms and that may be considered disruptive by some people. Parents of these children are often blamed for not being able to control their children properly in public, particularly since children with autism are phenotypically normal in appearance. Some of the societal reactions to families of children with developmental disabilities are explored more fully in Chapter 7.

A Note on Terminology

As we have seen, the terms used to refer to individuals with intellectual disabilities have evolved over the years. Recently, the American Association on Mental Retardation, an American professional organization founded in 1876, changed its name to the American Association on Intellectual and Developmental Disabilities. Schalock, Luckasson, and Shogren (2007) argued for the shift in terminology, acknowledging that although the newer term covers the same population as the older one, it is less offensive to persons with disabilities and more consistent with international terminology.

The shifts in terminology over the years have been guided by the recommendations of professional organizations with an eye toward adopting language that is both clear enough to be useful for professional purposes and sensitive to the needs of individuals with disabilities. A continual balance is sought between using terms that have similar meanings across settings and maintaining respect for persons with disabilities and their linguistic preferences.

In this volume, I refer to individuals with intellectual or developmental disabilities, even in discussions of earlier studies in which such individuals were identified as having mental retardation or other conditions. In particular, I refer to children with disabilities, rather than disabled children, to emphasize that persons with disabilities are not defined by these conditions. Rather, these conditions are only one aspect of their lives.

RELEVANT THEORETICAL PERSPECTIVES

This section examines some theoretical models within psychology that are applicable to families of children with developmental disabilities and have guided some of the research discussed in subsequent chapters.

Stress Models

Diathesis–stress models assert that individuals have predispositions for various conditions and that stress may actualize these predispositions (Zuckerman, 1999). Such models make two claims. First, some individuals may be especially vulnerable to depression, anger, and other problems. Second, prolonged or significant stress may turn preexisting vulnerabilities into actual behavioral disturbances. For example, Rademaker, van Zuiden, Vermetten, and Geuze (2011) suggested that trait neuroticism is a risk factor for posttraumatic stress disorder.

There are some important limitations to the diathesis–stress approach. Belsky and Pluess (2009) suggested that the evidence for differential susceptibility needed to be bolstered. They also argued that the model does not give sufficient attention to human plasticity—the ability of individuals to adjust well to their circumstances. Thus, the diathesis–stress model may assist researchers in understanding the risks, but not the potential for growth, for parents of children with special needs.

Nonetheless, the notion of predispositions may be useful in understanding the range of ways that families of children with developmental disabilities respond to the stresses they encounter. For example, as we shall see in Chapter 3, parents of children with developmental disabilities have an elevated risk of depressive symptoms. Diathesis–stress models may help explain why some but not all parents develop these symptoms. Recent research suggests that preexisting temperamental and behavioral characteristics of mothers of children with autism may interact with parenting stresses to lead to depressive symptoms.

Transactional Models

Transactional models capture the dynamic nature of human relationships (Sameroff, 2009). We all live in a social world, influenced by and influencing others around us. As one person changes, the surrounding individuals necessarily respond in some way. Transactional models are especially appropriate in understanding developmental change. Whereas many developmental models emphasize how parental behavior may shape child development, transactional models recognize that socialization is a bidirectional process and that children modify parental behaviors as well. An example of the transactional approach is the association between boys' conduct problems and mothers' depressive symptoms. Shaw, Gross, and Moilanen (2009) found that disruptive child behaviors at an early age predicted maternal depressive symptoms, which, in turn, were related to subsequent youth antisocial behavior as well as teacher reports of externalizing behaviors.

One transactional pattern that has been found in families of children with disabilities is overprotectiveness. Chapter 4 presents research suggesting that parents of children with developmental disabilities show higher levels of overprotectiveness than parents of more typically developing children. Studies of parents of children with spina bifida have found higher levels of overprotection than in the general population, and this form of parenting was associated with lower levels of behavioral autonomy in preadolescents with spina bifida, which was in turn associated with externalizing problems.

Ecological Models

Ecological models of development emphasize the role of context in human development. Ceci and Hembrooke (1995) suggested that many theories of development regard context as noise—that is, as a variable that needs to be controlled to understand the developmental process properly. In contrast,

Ceci and Hembrooke argued that development is inherently contextual, and thus one needs to appreciate the contexts of development to understand the developmental process. Although Ceci and Hembrooke identify several types of context, the social context is most relevant here.

Bronfenbrenner's (1977, 1999) bioecological model identified four levels of context that pertain to children's development. The *microsystem* context includes the immediate settings that children inhabit, such as the home, school, and neighborhood. The *mesosystem* context deals with the relationships between two or more microsystems; for example, interactions between parents and children in the home may influence a child's work at school, and vice versa. Next is the *exosystem* context, which refers to microsystems that do not contain the developing person but that may influence a child indirectly. For example, parental stresses at work may spill over into family life. Finally, there is the *macrosystem*, which includes large-scale social, economic, and political systems that can shape the daily lives of children. The macrosystem would include race and poverty as influential factors in a child's development.

More broadly, a concern for the environmental context draws our attention to broader cultural forces, including racial and ethnic issues that may affect the lives of children with disabilities. Studies suggest that there are disparities among black, Hispanic, and White children in their access to quality health care. Moreover, the challenges that parents face in collaborating with educators once their children enter the educational system may be greater for individuals who come from culturally or linguistically diverse groups.

The primary advantage of the ecological model for understanding families of children with disabilities is that it provides a broader perspective for understanding both areas of stress and opportunities for social support for such families. As children with disabilities enter the school system, for example, parents work to become partners with teachers, school psychologists, physical therapists, and other educational professionals to create an educational plan for their children. Often, such a plan requires coordination of therapy at school with therapy at home, which is an example of Bronfenbrenner's mesosystem context.

Positive Psychology Perspectives

Positive psychology emerged in the final years of the last millennium (Seligman & Csikszentmihalyi, 2000). The central claim of positive psychology is that psychology has focused too narrowly on pathology. Positive psychology emphasizes features that make life worth living, such as hope, wisdom, courage, and perseverance. It also examines questions such as what are the things that make people happy, how optimism affects a person's health, and what constitutes wisdom. Many of these traits and issues are relevant to the families of children with disabilities.

A key feature of positive psychology is the identification of character strengths. Several studies have converged on six core character strengths: wisdom and knowledge, courage, humanity, justice, temperance, and transcendence. N. Park, Peterson, and Seligman (2006) examined the prevalence of these character strengths in a large web-based study of 54 nations. They found significant commonalities across nations and across different regions of the United States, suggesting that there may be a set of universal character strengths. Moreover, Peterson, Park, Pole, D'Andrea, and Seligman (2008) found small but positive correlations between the number of traumatic events individuals experienced and increases in character strengths, suggesting that personal growth may follow the experience of trauma.

Although most of the literature on families of children with developmental disabilities emphasizes the stresses such families must contend with, a small but growing line of research indicates that parenting children with disabilities may contribute to personal growth. Parents sometimes adjust well to circumstances that they could not have anticipated and may report changes in spirituality, meaning, and values that they regard as positive.

Each of the four models discussed provides a useful framework for understanding families of children with developmental disabilities. The organization in this book is most obviously related to the transactional and ecological models. Early chapters focus on the initial experience of becoming a parent of a child with a special health care need, and subsequent chapters consider issues that emerge when individuals with disabilities reach childhood, adolescence, and early adulthood. These chapters explore how the nature of the transactions between parent and child evolves over time. Successive chapters examine different systems, including the family, the medical clinic, the school system, and society as a whole. Finally, the discussion throughout highlights the dual themes of stress and personal growth as they occur both over time and in various contextual systems.

METHODOLOGICAL CONSIDERATIONS

Stoneman (2007a) provided an overview of methodological issues associated with research on disabilities. One significant concern is the availability of families to study. Stoneman (2007a) noted that researchers generally do not have direct access to families who are receiving services and thus must depend on gatekeepers who screen families. This process, although necessary, may introduce bias. Gatekeepers may select families that they consider to be "good" participants likely to complete the study. Stoneman (2007a) reported that single parents, low-income families, and minority families were less likely to be informed of the opportunity to participate in research studies. As a consequence, our knowledge of these groups may be more limited; in particular, little research has examined the experience of a single parent with a child with a disability.

An additional consideration is the diversity of methodological approaches for studying disability and the consequent challenge of integrating these approaches into a coherent story. The study of children with developmental disabilities draws investigators from a wide variety of academic disciplines, including but not limited to psychology, special education, pediatrics, nursing, and sociology. Each of these disciplines brings insights into the experience of these families that complement the others and are needed for a fuller understanding of these families.

Disciplinary diversity brings methodological diversity. In the pages to follow, we consider randomized controlled experiments that compare the effectiveness of different treatment models for alleviating stress in families. Such studies are essential for gaining a clear understanding of how best to help these families, but other questions demand other approaches. For example, the study of communication between medical professionals and parents of children with disabilities requires an application of the methods of discourse analysis. Similarly, we will use qualitative analysis to understand narratives of parents of children with disabilities. In short, the topic at hand requires methodological pluralism.

OVERVIEW OF THE VOLUME

Chapter 2 examines how parents initially become aware that their child is "different" from their expectations. It discusses the stress associated with having an infant with significant medical concerns in the immediate postnatal period and the extent to which parents may suffer posttraumatic stress symptoms. Chapter 2 also introduces the secondary theme that different types of disabilities present distinct challenges to parents. For children with autism or cerebral palsy, the exact nature of the disability may be difficult to discern, and numerous medical appointments and a significant period of uncertainty may result. For other types of disabilities, such as Down syndrome, the diagnosis may be apparent at birth and confirmed shortly afterwards. The chapter discusses how diagnostic uncertainty may shape parental experience.

Chapter 3 considers the more enduring responses of parents to the stressors associated with having children with developmental or medical issues. The chapter reviews studies that examine the effects of different types of coping styles on perceived stress in parents of children with disabilities. It examines research suggesting that parents of children with disabilities may adjust well to their circumstances and connects these studies with the field of positive psychology.

Chapters 4 through 6 examine microsystems as contexts for family development. Chapter 4 discusses the family as a system and the notion that the introduction of a new family member leads to a new social organization. How parents balance work and family life and determine family roles when there is a child with a disability is discussed, and the experiences of siblings and grandparents are then considered. Chapters 5 and 6 look at family interaction with health care professionals and educational professionals, respectively. Chapter 5 discusses challenges in gaining access to medical care and equipment as well as the financial hardships associated with securing appropriate services. The chapter reviews the nature and impact of medical communication between parents and physicians. Chapter 6 compares and contrasts the attitudes of parents, teachers, and principals regarding the inclusion of children with disabilities in the general education classroom and discusses how some parents become advocates for their children's education and, more generally, for educational and societal change.

Chapter 7 discusses the macrosystem: how individuals with disabilities and their families are viewed in society. The perspectives of sociologists and social psychologists are used in discussing how individuals with disabilities are excluded from some social settings and the psychological impact of social exclusion. Chapter 7 also discusses the influence of informal social support such as parent support groups for families of children with disabilities.

Chapter 8 examines family changes as individuals with disabilities approach adolescence and early adulthood. It includes a discussion of the decision to place a child in a community living environment as well as employment issues for both parents and children. The chapter also addresses long-term relationships between individuals with disabilities and their adult siblings. Chapter 9 examines the implications of work on the narrative studies of lives for families touched by developmental disabilities. The chapter considers the extent to which family narratives emphasize themes that are congruent with those found in other narrative studies and the psychological consequences of different narrative strategies.

Various developmental disabilities are associated with a shorter life expectancy; as a consequence, the experience of losing a child with a disability may be a significant part of the overall parenting story. Chapter 10 discusses the varieties of bereavement responses when a child with a disability dies. This chapter reviews the scientific literature available on the variability of grief reactions and then examines the prominent themes in parents' responses to their children's death. It discusses how social constraints may interfere with a family's recovery from loss as well as the ways in which the life and death of a child with a developmental disability may be a meaningful life experience for parents.

Chapter 11 addresses clinical implications and begins by discussing the recent American Psychological Association (2012) guidelines for working with individuals and their families. Disability issues in the curricula of graduate programs in clinical psychology are discussed. The remainder of the chapter discusses randomized clinical trials that have assessed programs designed to reduce stress and increase happiness in families of children with developmental disorders.

Chapter 12 summarizes the major conclusions that may be drawn from current research literature. It identifies gaps in knowledge and suggests directions for future study.

2

INITIAL EXPERIENCE AND REACTIONS

I was scared; I could hardly breathe the first year. It was a terrible phase and that enormous feeling of loneliness—to be sent home from hospital with no one to contact. They could at least have given me a brochure or told me about a parental advocacy group, or something. It was so awful. (Gundersen, 2011, p. 86)

Parents learn of their child's diagnosis of a developmental disability in different ways. In some cases, the child is born premature or with low birth weight and requires immediate medical intervention. Medical staff may communicate concerns about the infant's development following the immediate medical crisis. In other cases, the child is apparently healthy at birth, and the parents come to understand the nature of the child's disability gradually over time. The differences in how parents learn of their child's disability may have a profound effect on how they respond in the immediate postnatal period as well as in the months and years to follow.

Infants who are premature or are low in birth weight are disproportionately likely to have developmental disabilities (Caravale, Tozzi, Albino, & Vicari, 2005; Marlow, Wolke, Bracewell, & Samara, 2005; McGowan, Alderdice, Holmes, & Johnston, 2011), so I begin with a discussion of the

http://dx.doi.org/10.1037/14192-002
Families of Children With Developmental Disabilities: Understanding Stress and Opportunities for Growth, by D. W. Carroll

experience of parents of premature and low birth weight infants. Later in the chapter, I consider some of the diverse ways in which parents receive a formal diagnosis of their child's condition and how they respond to these diagnoses.

IMMEDIATE PERINATAL EXPERIENCE

Newborn Intensive Care Unit

In most hospitals, infants born at biological risk, typically premature infants (less than 37-week gestational age) and infants with low birth weight (less than 2,500 grams), are ordinarily referred to the newborn intensive care unit (NICU) for further evaluation and treatment. The NICU is different from a typical infant nursery. Premature infants are usually attached to multiple monitors that track the infant's heartbeat, breathing, and the amount of oxygen in the blood. The baby may be attached to pumps that deliver medication and prevent dehydration. Some premature infants develop jaundice and are given phototherapy. Babies that have difficulty breathing may be placed on a ventilator.

The equipment may seem overwhelming to the new parents. One new parent of twins put it this way:

> They were so tiny, so still, so out of their element; hooked up to all kinds of wires, breathing machines, under bright lights with tiny masks over their eyes, wearing the tiniest little diapers that were still so big on them. It looked like something you would see on television, not something that would ever happen to your own babies. It was so surreal. I remember I felt so disconnected from them like they were not my babies, not my girls that were growing inside of me just a few short hours ago. (McDermott-Perez, 2007, p. 128[1])

In addition, parents quickly discover that their newborn will be attended to by a variety of medical specialists. The list begins with the child's pediatrician and, in many hospitals, a neonatologist who specializes in newborn intensive care. Other medical specialists may include nurse practitioners: physical, occupational, and respiratory therapists; and—depending on the infant's condition—cardiologists, neurologists, or gastroenterologists.

Parents of premature infants may be presented with some difficult cognitive tasks at a time when their physical and emotional resources are drained. They need to keep track of a variety of medical concerns and the medical team responsible for each one. They need to understand medical issues as they arise, and they may be required to make significant decisions regarding their infant's treatment shortly after the infant's birth.

---

[1]Passages in this chapter are from *Preemie Parents: Recovering From Baby's Premature Birth* (pp. 120–128), by L. McDermott-Perez, 2007, Westport, CT: Praeger. Copyright 2007 by Praeger. Reprinted with permission.

Immediate Stress Responses

The immediate responses of parents are consistent with Selye's (1976) description of the *general adaptation syndrome*. Selye suggested that humans or animals move through a general pattern in responding to heat, cold, noise, and other stressors. The general adaptation syndrome consists of three stages. In the first stage, alarm, the body responds immediately to the stressor. The second stage is resistance, in which there are declines in physical functioning with the persistence of a stressor. Finally, if the stressor continues after the individual's resources are depleted, a person moves into the exhaustion stage.

Parental reports in the first few days after their infant has been admitted into the NICU suggest an alarm response:

> Now that she had arrived, I had no time for depression. Or maybe it was simply my way of coping—in the midst of a crisis, hopelessness was a luxury I could not afford. Although I did not consciously make that decision, when I look back, I think my denial saved me. It kept me from falling apart when my baby needed me most. As the mother of a preemie, I had duties to attend to. (McDermott-Perez, 2007, p. 120)

Obeidat, Bond, and Callister (2009) reviewed 14 qualitative studies of parents' experience of having an infant in the NICU. Among the common responses were a sense of shock at the immediate crisis, grief at the loss of a dream, and the perception of being in an alien world.

Quantitative assessments of parent responses lead to similar conclusions. One of the most common tools for assessing parents' perception of stressors during the NICU period is the Parent Stressor Scale: Neonatal Intensive Care Unit (PSS:NICU) developed by Miles and Funk (1993). The instrument includes four dimensions: sights and sounds of the unit (e.g., monitors and equipment, sudden noises or alarms), infant behavior and appearance (e.g., small size, limpness), staff relationships (e.g., many different people, explaining things too quickly), and parental role alteration (e.g., difficulties in feeding, inability to hold infant). Parents rate each of the 46 items on a 1 to 5 scale. Miles, Funk, and Kasper (1991) found that alterations in parental role generated the highest level of stress, followed by infant behavior and appearance.

Maternal stress influences the initial interactions between mothers and their premature infants. In particular, it influences early feeding. Lau, Hurst, Smith, and Schanler (2007) compared stress responses and milk expression in African American, Caucasian, and Hispanic mothers. They investigated associations between psychosocial factors, frequency of milk expression, skin-to-skin holding, and lactation performance. Stress responses were similar in the three groups. On the PSS:NICU, the highest level of stress was recorded on the parental role alteration scale, which correlated negatively with the maternal drive to express milk.

Posttraumatic Stress Disorder

The impact of having an infant in the NICU is not necessarily limited to the short term. Some parents experience lingering effects that resemble posttraumatic stress disorder (PTSD). PTSD is recognized in the *Diagnostic and Statistical Manual of Mental Disorders* (4th ed., text rev.; *DSM-IV-TR*; American Psychiatric Association, 2000). PTSD is characterized by a variety of symptoms, including reliving of the traumatic event, avoidance of stimuli associated with the trauma, and high levels of emotional arousal.

The Perinatal Posttraumatic Stress Disorder Questionnaire (PPQ) is based on the diagnostic criteria for PTSD in the *DSM* (DeMier et al., 2000). It is a 14-item retrospective screening tool that asks parents of high-risk infants to assess the presence of traumatic recollections about delivery. Example items are "Did you have several bad dreams of giving birth or your baby's hospital stay?" and "Were you unable to remember parts of your baby's hospital stay?" Evidence indicates that PPQ scores are correlated with infant medical issues. Quinnell and Hynan (1999) found that mothers of high-risk infants scored higher than mothers of typically developing infants on the PPQ. DeMier et al. (2000) found that PTSD symptoms in mothers correlated with postnatal complications in their infants and with measures of infant maturity.

J. L. Callahan and Hynan (2002) evaluated the construct validity of the PPQ. Responses to four questionnaires by 121 high-risk and 52 low-risk mothers indicated that high-risk mothers showed higher levels of emotional distress on all measures. In addition, PPQ scores correlated positively with the tendency for mothers to seek formal psychotherapy for their childbirth experiences. Holditch-Davis et al. (2009) found correlations between parental stress, as measured by the PPQ, and measures of depression, state anxiety, posttraumatic stress, and daily hassles up to 24 months following the NICU experience. High levels of maternal stress were associated with higher levels of infant sickness and lower educational levels of mothers.

Several studies have explored the relationships between measures of posttraumatic stress and assessment of parent–child interaction and child development. Pierrehumbert, Nicole, Muller-Nix, Forcada-Guex, and Ansermet (2003) examined the role of parental posttraumatic reactions on sleeping and eating issues for their premature infants. Mothers and fathers of premature infants and a control group of parents with full-term infants were interviewed about eating and sleeping issues when their children were 18 months old, and parents completed the PPQ. Whereas only 6% of the control parents exhibited symptoms of PTSD, 67% of parents of premature infants exhibited such symptoms. Interestingly, the severity of the perinatal risks only partly predicted a child's problems; the intensity of the post-traumatic reactions of the parents, independent of perinatal risks, predicted these problems. Similarly, Muller-Nix et al. (2004) found that maternal stress as measured by the PPQ was positively correlated with disruptions in mother–infant interaction. At 6 months, mothers of high-risk infants were assessed to be less sensitive and more controlling.

Other measures have found converging results. Using the Impact of Events scale, a self-report measure designed to assess response to traumatic stressors, Åhlund, Clarke, Hill, and Thalange (2009) examined symptoms of PTSDs in mothers of very low birth weight infants 2 to 3 years postpartum. Compared with mothers of full-term, normal weight infants, mothers of infants with very low birth weight had significantly higher PTSD symptoms. Holditch-Davis, Bartlett, Blickman, and Miles (2003) conducted semistructured interviews with 30 mothers of high-risk premature infants at enrollment and when the infant was 6 months old, corrected for prematurity. All of the mothers experienced at least one posttraumatic symptom, 12 had two symptoms, and 16 had three symptoms. The most common reported symptoms were heightened arousal, reexperiencing of the premature birth, and avoidance. Garel, Dardennes, and Blondel (2007) assessed maternal distress 1 year after preterm childbirth using a qualitative methodology. Semistructured interviews indicated that most of the mothers experienced fatigue, depression, guilt, and anxiety regarding their experience, and some indicated that they tried to avoid thinking about the birth, but that was impossible. Maternal reports of their child's behavior and their own health were more negative at 1 year than at 2 months after discharge.

In sum, research studies suggest that being a parent of an infant in a NICU may lead to significant long-term symptoms similar to PTSD. The stress responses may disrupt mother–child interaction and lead to sleeping and eating issues. The stress may be partly due to the severity of the child's health issues, but the parental perception of stress, independent of the infant's health status, is an important predictor of long-term emotional distress in the parent. The extent to which PTSD symptoms are related to preexisting issues, such as parental anxiety or marital quality, has not been adequately investigated.

Intervention Programs

Studies discussed in the previous section suggest that parental response to premature birth mediates later adverse child outcomes related to sleeping and feeding. Thus, parental response should be a target of intervention efforts. Intervention programs have been focused on reducing parental stress, increasing parental skills in responding to their infants, increasing parental knowledge, or a combination of these approaches. Jotzo and Poets (2005) examined the effectiveness of a trauma-prevention program during hospitalization for parents of premature infants. Mothers of premature infants were enrolled consecutively in a sequential control group design. Intervention group mothers received a structured psychological intervention in the first days after birth and were actively approached at critical times during their infant's NICU stay. The intervention included both educational and relaxation components. Control mothers did not receive psychological intervention but could ask for counseling by the hospital minister. At discharge, intervention group mothers showed significantly lower levels of traumatic response than the control group: Nineteen mothers in the control group showed symptoms of clinically significant psychological trauma, compared with nine in the intervention group.

Melnyk, Crean, Feinsein, and Fairbanks (2008) examined whether an educational–behavioral intervention program influenced maternal anxiety and depression following premature infants' discharge from the NICU. Measures included the PSS:NICU, the State–Trait Anxiety Inventory, and the Beck Depression Inventory. A measure of mother–infant interaction and a measure of mothers' beliefs about their infant and role were also included. Mothers were assessed 2 months following infant discharge. Mothers were randomly assigned to treatment or control groups. The treatment program provided parents with information on the appearance and behavioral characteristics of premature infants and how parents can participate in their infants' care as well as with information on activities that assist parents in identifying infant stress cues. The researchers found that the intervention program lessened postdischarge maternal anxiety and depression.

Browne and Talmi (2005) examined how family-based interventions may increase parental knowledge and decrease stress. The researchers randomly assigned 84 high-risk mother–infant dyads to two intervention groups and one control group. One group participated in a demonstration of infant reflexes, attention, motor skills, and sleep–wake states. A second group viewed educational materials. A third group, serving as a control, participated in an informal discussion. Mothers in both intervention groups showed greater knowledge of infant behavior and more sensitive interactions with their infants shortly after discharge.

These intervention programs, although effective, are primarily directed at immediate issues. However, the link between parental stress and PTSD suggests that longer-term programs may also be beneficial. In Chapter 11, I examine programs to assist parents of children with developmental disabilities who have more enduring psychological needs.

PARENTAL RESPONSES TO CHILD DIAGNOSIS

Parental Uncertainty and Information Seeking

One of the needs that parents often experience in the first days after the birth of a preterm child or a child with health issues is simply to better understand the nature of the infant's problems. Cacioppo, Petty, Feinstein, and Jarvis (1996) reviewed the literature on the *need for cognition*, defined as an individual's motivation to engage in effortful cognitive endeavors. Much of the literature emphasizes that the need for cognition differs significantly between individuals. For example, some people appear to have a higher level of causal uncertainty than others, and this attribute is positively correlated with depressive symptoms (Weary & Edwards, 1994). Weary and Jacobson (1997) provided support for the assertion that causal uncertainty beliefs lead to diagnostic information seeking.

Graungaard and Skov (2007) reported that uncertainty is a major issue for parents of children with disabilities. They conducted a qualitative, longitudinal study using interviews of 16 parents whose children had recently been diagnosed as having physical or mental disabilities. The results indicated that parents were distressed by the uncertainty associated with their child's diagnosis, felt powerless, and wanted to know what they could do to help their child. Pain (1999) conducted semistructured interviews with parents of children with disabilities to determine what information they had learned about their children's disabilities and how helpful the information was. The research found that information helped parents to adjust emotionally to their child's disabilities, to access services and benefits, and to improve their management of the child's behavior. For the most part, parents found information to be useful.

Some studies of the ability of parents to "resolve" the loss or trauma associated with their child's diagnosis have been undertaken with an instrument called the Reactions to Diagnosis Interview (RDI). Trained interviewers ask parents questions designed to elicit strategies for dealing with the diagnosis, including a reorientation to the present, a realistic view of the child, a termination of the search for existential reasons for the child's condition (i.e., "Why did this happen to me?"), and a balanced view of the impact of their experience on their lives. Videotaped interviews are then analyzed into various categories.

Studies of the RDI indicate that resolution of diagnosis is related to parental adjustment. Sheeran, Marvin, and Pianta (1997) investigated the relationship between mothers' resolution of their child's diagnosis and self-reported parenting stress, marital quality, and social support in mothers of children with cerebral palsy or epilepsy. Mothers categorized as resolved reported less parenting stress, greater satisfaction with their husbands, and higher levels of helpful family support. Lord, Ungerer, and Wastell (2008) found that 69% of mothers and 77% of fathers of children with phenylketonuria were resolved to their child's diagnosis, and that parental resolution was positively correlated with parental adjustment.

Role of Diagnostic Categories

An early approach to conceptualizing parental responses to child diagnosis was the chronic sorrow hypothesis (Olshansky, 1962). The suggestion was that parents of children with developmental disabilities struggled to cope with the loss of a "perfect child." Olshansky (1962) characterized chronic sorrow as the normal response to an event that violated parental expectations. Subsequent research has found that parental responses include not only sorrow but also fear, helplessness, anger, frustration, and other aspects of grief (Eakes, Burke, & Hainsworth, 1998).

Rather than emphasizing, as the chronic sorrow hypothesis does, a "one-size-fits-all" approach, it may be more profitable to see parental responses to diagnosis as more diverse and variable. In particular, parental responses may be related to the diagnosis they are presented with, along with when they are presented with it. The clearest data we have are from parents of children diagnosed with Down syndrome, autism, and cerebral palsy.

Down Syndrome

Down syndrome is typically diagnosed quickly. The facial characteristics of Down syndrome may be apparent at birth, and the syndrome can be confirmed quickly and authoritatively through genetic tests. Devlin and Morrison (2004) reported that 89% of the cases of Down syndrome they studied were diagnosed between one and seven days of life. Given the typically early and definitive diagnosis, we might expect parental adjustment to a child with Down syndrome to be somewhat easier than for a parent facing greater uncertainty.

Some evidence bears on this issue. Lenhard et al. (2005) studied mothers of children with Down syndrome, mothers of children with intellectual disabilities of uncertain origin, and mothers of children without disabilities. They compared the three groups on measures of anxiety, guilt, and emotional strain. Mothers of children with unknown diagnoses had significantly higher levels of anxiety, regret, and emotional stress than mothers of children without disabilities. Mothers of children with Down syndrome had responses similar to those of mothers of children without disabilities on most measures, although they did report more regret for having more problems than other parents. These results suggest that diagnostic certainty may alleviate stress in mothers of children with disabilities. When mothers have a name for a condition, they may be better able to access different forms of support, such as online resources and parent support groups. In this context, it is noteworthy that the mothers of children with Down syndrome were much more likely (34.8%) to have joined a self-help group than were mothers of children with unknown etiology (14.0%) or mothers of children without disabilities (4.4%). It is likely that the self-help group, in addition to the clear diagnosis, contributed to these mothers' well-being.

Other studies have found converging results (Carroll, 2009; Perry, Harris, & Minnes, 2004). Perry et al. (2004) studied mothers and fathers with children with one of five types of developmental disability: Down syndrome, fragile X syndrome (FXS), Rett syndrome, autism, and developmental disability of unknown etiology. The researchers found that parents of children with Down syndrome scored significantly higher on a measure of family harmony than did parents of children with unknown etiology. Family harmony scores were intermediate for families of children with FXS, Rett syndrome, and autism.

Autism Spectrum Disorder

In contrast to Down syndrome, autism spectrum disorder (including autism, Asperger's syndrome, and pervasive developmental disorder—not otherwise specified) is typically diagnosed much later than other developmental disabilities. Although diagnosis as early as 2 or 3 years of age has been reported (Charman & Baird, 2002), most studies suggest that the diagnosis is made around 4 or 5 years of age (Goin-Kochel, Mackintosh, & Myers, 2006; Shattuck et al., 2009). Newschaffer et al. (2007) reported that there are often significant delays between initial parent concerns and formal diagnosis; the lag in diagnosis may be shorter if there is family history of autism (Ozonoff et al., 2009).

Autism spectrum disorder is diagnosed relatively slowly for several reasons: As it is currently understood, it consists of a spectrum of loosely related disorders differing in severity. The diagnostic criteria for these disorders are less clear-cut than for Down syndrome. Shifts in diagnostic criteria have also contributed to confusion regarding the incidence of autism spectrum disorder. Epidemiological surveys indicate that the estimated prevalence of the disorder increased from approximately four in 10,000 in the mid-1960s to as high as 60 in 10,000 in some estimates by 2001 (Fombonne, 2003). The current estimate is one in 88 (Centers for Disease Control and Prevention, 2012). Gernsbacher, Dawson, and Goldsmith (2005) argued that no sound scientific evidence existed to indicate that there is an increase in the incidence of autism. To the contrary, they suggested that the increase in reported cases is merely due to intentionally broadened diagnostic criteria.

In support of this contention, Shattuck (2006) observed that the increased diagnosis of autism had been accompanied by a decrease in diagnosis of related conditions. Fombonne, Zakarian, Bennett, Meng, and McLean-Heywood (2006) agreed, suggesting that changes in definition along with improved awareness explain much of the upward trend in recent decades. Similarly, M. King and Bearman (2009) estimated that perhaps one in four children diagnosed with autism today would not have received the diagnosis in 1993.

In addition, media coverage of speculations regarding the cause of autism has contributed to parental uncertainty. In particular, considerable coverage has concerned the possible role of vaccines in the presumed epidemic. Although the scientific community initially supported the hypothesis that autism was linked causally to vaccines, the research has been retracted (Murch et al., 2004).

It is also likely that public attitudes toward different disabilities play a role here, in that some individuals may perceive fewer stigmas attached to autism than to mild intellectual disabilities. Moreover, diagnostic trends may be influenced by changes in the rates of funding for services for different conditions in various locales (Nassar et al., 2009).

As a consequence of these factors, diagnoses of autism spectrum disorder are made much later than diagnoses of Down syndrome. We might thus expect that confusion regarding diagnosis may complicate parental resolution. Although no studies have directly compared parents of children with autism and Down syndrome, several studies suggest that resolution levels are relatively low for parents of children with autism. Milshtein, Yirmiya, Oppenheim, Koren-Karie, and Levi (2010) interviewed parents of children with autism spectrum disorder (mean age = 8.1 years) and found that slightly less than half of the parents in their study were identified as resolved. Mothers were more likely to be unresolved whereas fathers were evenly split. Oppenheim, Koren-Karie, Dolev, and Yirmiya (2009) found similar results in somewhat younger children (mean age = 49 months).

The lag between initial parental concerns and diagnosis of autism spectrum disorder (ASD) may be greater for families from minority communities. Mandell, Listerud, Levy, and Pinto-Martin (2002) examined racial disparities in the timing of the diagnosis of ASD. Age of diagnosis was significantly earlier for White children (6.3 years) than for Black children (7.9 years). In a subsequent study, Mandell et al. (2009) examined records of children who met the diagnostic criteria for ASD even if they had not received a documented diagnosis. They reported that Black and Hispanic children were less likely to be recognized as ASD as White children.

In addition, socioeconomic factors appear to influence diagnosis of ASD. Mandell, Novak, and Zubritsky (2005) found few racial differences in the timing of diagnosis, but the age of diagnosis was later for poorer children and children from rural areas. Fountain, King, and Bearman (2011) also found that the timing of ASD diagnosis was related to socioeconomic status factors. Mandell and Novak (2005) suggested that observed disparities in the timing of diagnoses might reflect broader cultural disparities in access to health care (to be discussed in Chapter 5). For a review of issues pertaining to the diagnosis and treatment of ASD, see Shattuck and Grosse (2007).

Some studies have examined correlates of parental resolution. Goin-Kochel et al. (2006) studied parents of children diagnosed with autism, Asperger's syndrome, or pervasive developmental disorder. Higher levels of parental education and income were associated with earlier diagnosis and greater satisfaction with the diagnostic process. In addition, parents were more satisfied with the diagnostic process when they required fewer appointments with professionals to get the diagnosis and when the children received the diagnosis at younger ages. Dale, Jahoda, and Knott (2006) examined maternal attributions following their child's diagnosis with autism. Although the attributions were diverse, they reflected the uncertainty regarding cause and prognosis. Mothers who felt they had no control over helping their child had higher levels of depressive symptoms.

Although parents of children with autism have relatively low levels of resolution as measured by the RDI, those who achieve resolution have better well-being. Milshtein et al. (2010) found that maternal (but not paternal) resolution status was associated with reported negative impact of raising a child with a disability on family life. Unresolved mothers had significantly higher negative feelings about parenting and expressed greater concern for the impact of the child's disability on their marriage. Wachtel and Carter (2008) found that mothers who were more emotionally resolved were rated as higher in cognitive and supportive engagement in play interactions with their children. Moreover, Oppenheim et al. (2009) found that mothers of preschoolers with ASD who had resolved their child's diagnosis were more likely to have children who were securely attached. These and other investigators suggested that parental resolution should be a target for intervention efforts.

Other Developmental Disabilities

Down syndrome and autism provide the clearest contrast, but there are a handful of studies of other syndromes. I. Rentinck, Ketelaar, Jongmans, Lindeman, and Gorter (2009) found that about three quarters of parents of children diagnosed with cerebral palsy were identified on the RDI as resolved by 18 months of age. Similarly, Schuengel et al. (2009) found that more than

80% of parents of children with cerebral palsy indicated resolution. Unresolved reactions were more often found among parents of younger children and parents of children with more severe motor disabilities. For parents of younger children, resolution often took the form of constructive thoughts and information seeking. In a longitudinal study, I. C. M. Rentinck et al. (2010) found considerable stability in the resolution status of parents; 82% of parents were identified as resolved when the child was 18 months of age, and 1 year later the percentage increased to 89%. Although these results suggest that resolution in parents of children with cerebral palsy is relatively stable, I. C. M. Rentinck et al. (2010) also noted that resolved parents may shift over time from a thinking-oriented strategy to an action-oriented strategy. Thus, even for "resolved" parents, resolution is an ongoing process.

Delays in diagnosis have been found for other conditions. Bailey, Skinner, and Sparkman (2003) surveyed 274 families who had at least one child with FXS to determine their experiences with diagnosis. Families reported several barriers to discovering FXS and frustration with the process. On average, the family expressed concern about the child's development at an average age of 13 months, but professional confirmation of developmental delay did not occur until 21 months and diagnosis of FXS at about 32 months. Similarly, Stochholm, Juul, Juel, Naeraa, and Gravholt (2006) reported wide variations in the age of diagnosis of Turner syndrome. Approximately 15% of individuals were diagnosed in the first year, one third during adolescence, and more than 38% in adulthood. The median age of diagnosis of Turner syndrome was 15.1 years.

Although most of the literature supports the notion that parents prefer and respond well to a clear diagnosis, Whitmarsh, Davis, Skinner, and Bailey (2007) presented a complementary view. Whitmarsh et al. found evidence that parents sometimes appreciate uncertainty. The researchers interviewed parents and grandparents of children with Klinefelter syndrome, Turner syndrome, and FXS to determine how they interpreted a confirmed genetic diagnosis that was associated with a range of possible symptoms. Parents viewed the genetic diagnosis as stable, permanent, and authoritative. However, some of the parents allowed, and even embraced, uncertainty about the condition by focusing on the variation between diagnosed siblings and the individuality of the disabled child. Other parents discounted the validity of the genetic diagnosis in the absence of current symptoms. This study provides an interesting and informative contrast with much of the literature. The authors suggest that parents of children with disabilities recognize both the values and drawbacks of diagnostic labels. On the one hand, such labels may be useful for qualifying a child for special services or for obtaining medical insurance. On the other hand, diagnostic labels may appear to provide greater certainty than is warranted for a particular child.

When that certainty is of a delayed developmental outcome, parents may prefer uncertainty.

For now, a preliminary conclusion is warranted: The experience of parents of children with Down syndrome, autism, and cerebral palsy differ at the outset. Down syndrome may be diagnosed relatively early and definitively. ASDs are typically diagnosed much later and exhibit a significant amount of intragroup variation. Cerebral palsy appears to be intermediate both in terms of the speed and definitiveness of the diagnosis. Parents of children with Down syndrome tend to resolve the diagnosis sooner than parents of children with autism, with parents of children with cerebral palsy again intermediate. For all groups, parental resolution is associated with family well-being.

These observations accord with what Hodapp, Ly, Fidler, and Ricci (2001) referred to as the *Down syndrome advantage*. Hodapp and colleagues observed that parents of children with Down syndrome reported less stress and more child-related rewards than parents of children with other disabilities. Subsequent work suggested that this advantage might be at least partially attributable to variance in family income (Stoneman, 2007b).

The observation that parental responses to diagnosis predict adjustment carries implications for intervention. Barnett, Clements, Kaplan-Estrin, and Fialka (2003) suggested that interventions may help parents adapt to their children by assisting them in developing new dreams for their children. The researchers presented a plan for a group intervention program to assist parents in identifying the range of feelings elicited by children with special needs, encouraging mutual support among parents, and improving skills at seeking information. At present, no research has been undertaken on the efficacy of intervention programs for modifying the immediate parental response to child diagnosis. It would be useful to understand the kinds of interventions that would be most helpful for parents of children with unclear diagnoses. Studies along this line may help in identifying ways in encouraging adaptive parental responses as early as possible, for the well-being of all members of the family.

To sum up, the initial experiences of parents of children with developmental disabilities vary with the nature of the disability and when it is diagnosed. Nonetheless, there are commonalities across disabilities: Parents face an uncertain future that they have not prepared for and must devote considerable personal resources to deal with the immediate crisis of having a child with significant if often poorly understood medical issues. The long-term consequences of the immediate crisis may be seen in posttraumatic symptoms several years later.

For parents of children who have enduring developmental issues, this is only the beginning. In the next chapter, I examine how parents begin to make longer-term adaptations in light of their child's development.

3

STRESS, COPING, AND GROWTH

I knew her condition was serious and her prognosis poor but, to me, she was my firstborn, beautiful child. Every time I expressed my joy to the staff at the hospital, they said, "She's denying reality." I understood the reality of my child's situation but, for me, there was another reality. (Kearney & Griffin, 2001, p. 583)

We saw in Chapter 2 how parents respond when confronted with the immediate crisis of a premature birth or the initial diagnosis of a developmental disability. Parents mobilize their resources to deal with the crisis, sometimes in ways that may influence them emotionally for years. However, when children have persistent developmental issues, parents must develop strategies for the long haul. In this chapter, I consider more enduring responses to the stresses associated with having a child with a developmental disability, with an emphasis on adaptations that occur during the preschool and early school years.

The first section of this chapter examines how stress affects parents and discusses the relationship between parenting stress and depression. It also considers variables, such as optimism and cognitive appraisal, that may moderate this relationship. The second section explores the notion that parenting a child with a developmental disability may promote personal growth. The chapter closes with a consideration of the mix of positive and negative emotions in parents of children with disabilities.

http://dx.doi.org/10.1037/14192-003
Families of Children With Developmental Disabilities: Understanding Stress and Opportunities for Growth,
by D. W. Carroll

STRESS AND COPING

Parenting Stress

Several studies have compared stress in parents of children with disabilities and parents of typically developing children. For example, Florian and Findler (2001) examined mental health and marital adaptation among 80 mothers of children with cerebral palsy and 80 mothers of typically developing children. The two groups were matched on demographic characteristics such as the number of children in the family, child gender, and maternal age. Florian and Findler found that mothers of children with cerebral palsy reported a significantly higher number of stressful life events and significantly lower levels of mental health and marital adaptation. Similar results have been found for other developmental disabilities such as autism (N. O. Davis & Carter, 2008), attention-deficit/hyperactivity disorder (Anastopolous, Guevremont, Shelton, & DuPaul, 1992), and fragile X syndrome (Johnston et al., 2003). Although there are occasional exceptions (e.g., Dyson, 1997), most studies have found significantly higher levels of stress in parents of children with disabilities.

One factor related to the level of parenting stress is child behavior. Lecavalier, Leone, and Wiltz (2006) studied parents of 293 young people with autism spectrum disorder (ASD). Parents completed measures of stress, behavior problems, social competence, and children's adaptive behavior. The researchers found that children's externalizing behaviors, especially conduct problems, were a significant predictor of stress. The data were consistent with a transactional model in which child behavior problems and parental stress exacerbated each other over time.

Several studies have emphasized the importance of social support in moderating the level of parenting stress. Plant and Sanders (2007) found that child problem behaviors and the difficulty of the caregiving task were strongly associated with parenting stress; level of disability had a lesser effect on stress. Moreover, the level of partner or family support moderated the relationships between these variables and parent stress. Similarly, in a study of 880 families of children with disabilities, T. B. Smith, Oliver, and Innocenti (2001) found that social support predicted parenting stress better than did aspects of child functioning.

Parental Stress and Depression

Several scholars have expressed interest in the relationship between having a child with a disability and parental depression. Considerable research suggests that parents of children with disabilities are more at risk for depressive symptoms. Manuel, Naughton, Balkrishnan, Smith, and Koman (2003) studied 270 mothers of children with cerebral palsy and found that 30% had depressive symptoms. Singer (2006) conducted a meta-analysis of 18 studies between 1984 and 2003. Results showed an elevated level of depressive symptoms in mothers of children with disabilities relative to those with children who were developing typically. Almost one third (29%) of the mothers in these studies experienced depression. Age of the child and disability category moderated the effect sizes.

The distinction between depressive symptoms and clinically diagnosed depression is important. Bailey, Golden, Roberts, and Ford (2007) critiqued the literature on maternal depression and developmental disability. Although the authors acknowledged that mothers of children with disabilities exhibited an elevated rate of depressive symptoms relative to the general population, they concluded that the incidence rate might be lower than reported in the literature due to measurement issues. In particular, most studies had relied on paper-and-pencil self-ratings that were not diagnostic clinical tools rather than on diagnoses by trained psychologists. They estimated that slightly less than 25% of mothers exhibit depressive symptoms, which was less than published reports, albeit slightly higher than the community-based rate.

Some efforts have been made to compare depressive symptoms across disabilities. As we have seen, the presence of a definitive diagnosis can assist parental adjustment to a child's disability. Feldman et al. (2007) compared Beck Depression Inventory (BDI) scores for primary caregivers (mainly biological mothers) of children with low birth weight or prematurity, children with known diagnoses (e.g., Down syndrome, spina bifida), and children with disabilities with unknown reasons. The latter group had the highest BDI scores. Child behavior problems were associated with caregiver depressive symptoms, but social support mediated and (partly) moderated this relationship. Singer (2006) found elevated rates of depression in mothers of children with autism relative to those with children with spina bifida or intellectual disabilities, suggesting that the additional services often required by such children may influence maternal well-being.

In a series of studies, Glidden and colleagues compared adoptive and birth mothers of children with intellectual disabilities. Glidden and Schoolcraft (2003) explored the trajectory of symptoms of depression in mothers of a child with a disability. Both adoptive and birth mothers reported low levels of depression. Glidden and Jobe (2006) extended these results, finding that adoptive mothers showed low levels of depression at the time of adoption and thereafter, whereas birth mothers showed significantly higher levels when their children were first diagnosed, but not at later times. However, mothers who had relatively high depression earlier still reported higher depression after 17 years.

In some recent and interesting work, Ingersoll and colleagues (Ingersoll & Hambrick, 2011; Ingersoll, Meyer, & Becker, 2011) examined the personal characteristics of mothers of children with and without ASD. In particular, the researchers examined the *broader autism phenotype* (BAP), which is a measure of subclinical personality and other features believed to index familiality or genetic liability to ASD. Mothers of children with ASD reported higher parenting stress and greater depressed mood than mothers of children without ASD. For mothers of children with ASD, BAP predicted the number of reported depressive symptoms, even after controlling for the severity of child autism and parenting stress. Ingersoll et al. (2011) found that two aspects of BAP—social skills and communication—best distinguished between mothers of children with ASD and mothers of children without ASD. The authors concluded that the elevated rate of depression in mothers of children with ASD might be attributable to the combined effect of high levels of parenting stress and personality features that placed mothers at higher risk for developing depression.

Regardless of the causes, depressive symptoms influence parenting quality. For example, depressive symptoms often produce lethargy, which can interfere with a person's willingness to make constructive adaptations to their current circumstances. As Featherstone (1981) observed, parents of children with disabilities are often fatigued by the multiple demands on their time, and such fatigue may lessen their willingness to consider changes in their lives, even changes that would improve their lives. Change requires effort, and a person who is truly tired may not be able to summon up the effort.

Optimism as a Moderator Variable

Gillham, Shatte, Reivich, and Seligman (2001) reviewed studies of optimism and pessimism as explanatory styles. *Explanatory style* refers to the characteristic ways that an individual explains good and bad events. Most research on explanatory style emphasizes three dimensions. *Internality* refers to whether a person attributes an event to an internal (i.e., personal) or external (i.e., environmental) cause. *Stability* refers to whether the cause is regarded as stable or transient. *Globality* refers to whether the attribution is a characteristic feature of a person's explanatory style or is merely a characteristic of one domain.

A pessimistic explanatory style is characterized by the tendency to attribute negative events to internal, stable, and global factors. Thus, when a person fails at a given task, the person may conclude that he or she is not intelligent enough to succeed. Conversely, positive events are attributed to external, temporary, and specific factors; for example, an unexpected good performance is attributed to dumb luck. This pattern of causal attributions diminishes future motivation (Dweck & Leggett, 1988) because it encourages a person to view events as uncontrollable. In contrast, optimism is an explanatory style that attributes negative events to external, transient, and specific factors. An optimistic person might explain a failed relationship as due to the strains that the two individuals had experienced recently at work, as opposed to more fundamental or enduring personal characteristics. Conversely, such a person views positive events as due to internal, stable, and global factors.

Questions arise regarding the application of these concepts to parents of children with developmental disabilities. How optimistic are the parents? What is the effect of optimism on reported parenting stress? Does optimism have a downside?

Several studies indicate that parents of children with developmental disabilities display high levels of optimism. Heiman (2002) interviewed 32 parents regarding their past, present, and future modes of coping. Although parents expressed high levels of frustration and dissatisfaction in attempting to maintain a routine life, the majority also expressed the need for a strong belief in the child and in the child's future, an optimistic outlook, and a realistic acceptance of the disability. Other studies (Kearney & Griffin, 2001; G. King, Baxter, Rosenbaum, Zwaigenbaum, & Bates, 2009) have also highlighted the importance of optimism in parents' reports of their experiences.

Optimism may moderate the relationship between parenting stress and health—both physical and psychological. B. L. Baker, Blacher, and Olsson (2005) found that parents of delayed and nondelayed preschoolers did not differ on depression or marital adjustment, but child behavior problems were strongly related to scores on both measures. Optimism moderated this relationship, primarily for mothers. When child behavior problems were high, mothers who were less optimistic received lower scores on measures of well-being than did mothers who were more optimistic. Similarly, Paczkowski and Baker (2008) examined the effect of positive beliefs on stress in parents of developmentally delayed and typically developing children at 3, 5, and 7 years of age. Positive beliefs moderated the effect of child behavior issues on parenting stress, at least for mothers of 3-year-olds.

In addition to moderating the effects of stressful events such as child behavior, optimism may serve as a mediator. Ekas, Lickenbrock, and Whitman (2010) studied the relationship between social support and maternal well-being. Family support was associated with increased optimism that, in turn, was correlated with higher levels of positive affect and life satisfaction as well as with lower levels of depression and parenting stress.

Thus, on the whole, optimism has primarily positive effects on the well-being of parents of children with disabilities. Nonetheless, Peterson and Vaidya (2003) have argued that optimism can have costs if it is too unrealistic. Although optimism may improve mood, health, and social relations, it may also encourage maladaptive persistence. In this light, S. E. Taylor (1989) drew a distinction between illusions (which are resistant to, but ultimately accommodate to, reality) and delusions (which do not). Although the tendency to see oneself in the best possible light is a sign of well-being, people also need to appraise their circumstances realistically.

The multiple uncertainties that parents of children with disabilities face—their child's prognosis, longevity, and future needs, among many others—raise questions about maladaptive persistence in parents. Some medical professionals who serve children with disabilities believe that some parents retain a higher level of hope than is realistic given their circumstances and push for aggressive therapies that have little chance of success (Baergen, 2006; Reder & Serwint, 2009; for a different view, see Hartshorne, 2002). There are no easy answers here. Optimism may be a critical coping strategy for a parent surrounded by challenges for the foreseeable future, but one that might have to bend to reality over time.

Cognitive Appraisal

Another psychological variable that has been considered as a moderator of the relationship between parenting stress and depressive symptoms is cognitive appraisal. Cognitive appraisal refers to the manner in which individuals interpret the events they experience, which is often related to their emotional reactions. Lazarus and Folkman (1984) distinguished between *problem-focused coping* and *emotion-focused coping*. Problem-focused coping addresses the problem that is causing personal distress, whereas emotion-focused coping may involve seeking emotional support or otherwise reducing emotional distress. More recently, Folkman and Moskowitz (2000) have examined *positive reappraisal*, which refers to cognitive strategies that reframe an event in a positive light. Positive reappraisal has been linked with positive affect during stressful events. Folkman and Moskowitz (2000) suggest that positive reappraisal may be especially helpful in assisting people who must sustain caregiving efforts over a long period of time.

Trute and colleagues examined parental appraisals of the family impact of a child with a disability. Trute and Hiebert-Murphy (2002) created a 15-item scale that assesses parental appraisal of the family implications of raising a child with a developmental disability. The scale included both positive (e.g., helping parents reassess their values) and negative (e.g., having to postpone family events) appraisals. The authors found that the net appraisal score predicted future parenting stress, even when other relevant variables (e.g., marital adjustment, level of disability) were statistically controlled.

Trute, Hiebert-Murphy, and Levine (2007) examined differences between mothers and fathers in their appraisals of child behavior. A total of 103 mothers and 55 fathers independently completed interviews at two points: 6 months after their child entered childhood disability services and 1 year later. Fathers had a lower level of positive appraisal at 6 months, suggesting that mothers formed positive affective ties to their children more quickly than fathers. However, gender differences in appraisal merged over time; no significant differences between mothers and fathers were observed at 1 year.

In addition, long-term family adjustment was predicted by the level of parental negative appraisal of the family and by level of self-esteem for both mothers and fathers. For mothers, positive appraisal of childhood disability was also found to predict early family adjustment and was related to enhanced self-esteem.

Conceptual Models

Several conceptual models have been proposed to summarize the existing literature with regard to the effects of stress on families and to guide future areas of exploration. The *double ABCX model* of family stress and adaptation (Lavee, McCubbin, & Patterson, 1985) has been influential. The model suggests that family stress (X) is influenced by a stressor (A), by the family's resources for dealing with the stressor (B), and by the family's perception of the stressor (C). In applications to families of children with disabilities, the stressor is a set of changing conditions associated with the child's disability. Resources include personal resources (e.g., knowledge, skills), family system resources (i.e., cohesion), and social support. Perception may include such factors as optimism, resilience, and locus of control. Lavee et al. (1985) provided evidence that the accumulation of events leads to family strain and that family system and social support moderate these relationships in different ways: family system variables influence the ability of families to adapt to changing demands, whereas social support serves as a buffer against stress.

K. A. Crnic, Friedrich, and Greenberg (1983) presented another influential model. Noting that research on children with disabilities to that point often produced inconsistent or contradictory findings, K. A. Crnic et al. suggested that an overly narrow focus on mothers and on negative outcomes was preventing researchers from understanding the full range of family responses to a child with a disability. Taking a family systems approach, K. A. Crnic et al. proposed a model that considered fathers and siblings in addition to mothers. They examined both positive and negative family adaptations of having a child with a disability. The model took an ecological approach in discussing the interrelationships between the family system and other social institutions such as the school environment.

Long before the positive psychology movement emerged, K. A. Crnic et al. (1983) drew attention to the finding that families of children with disabilities may experience positive as well as negative adaptations. I now turn to research examining whether positive outcomes for parents and family members follow a child's disability.

TRAUMATIC EXPERIENCE AND PERSONAL GROWTH

Although the majority of research on parenting children with disabilities has focused on the extent and nature of negative outcomes, indications of positive outcomes are scattered throughout the literature. The field of positive psychology (Seligman & Csikszentmihalyi, 2000) provides a useful conceptual framework for interpreting these outcomes.

Strength of Character and Posttraumatic Growth

Calhoun and Tedeschi (2001) discussed the positive lessons of loss. Reviewing studies of individuals who have experienced many different forms of traumatic loss (e.g., motorcycle accidents, breast cancer, death of a child, intense military combat), Calhoun and Tedeschi found evidence for changes in the individual's sense of self, changes in relationships, and spiritual growth. The authors reminded us that the presence of growth does not entail the absence of pain and distress. To the contrary, individuals with posttraumatic growth acknowledged both positive and negative aspects of their experiences.

Peterson, Park, Pole, D'Andrea, and Seligman (2008) researched how traumatic experiences may spur personal growth. Their web-based sample consisted of 1,739 adults who had experienced traumatic events such as a life-threatening accident or unwanted sexual contact under force or had witnessed someone being killed. At least one such event was reported by 56% of the sample, and 32% reported two or more. The researchers found a small but significant statistical association between traumatic events and increases in character strengths such as courage, kindness, creativity, and honesty. Individuals who reported a greater number of traumatic events showed greater increases in the character strengths.

Linley and Joseph (2004) reviewed 39 empirical studies of positive change following trauma and found that problem-focused coping, optimism, and positive affect were all consistently associated with adversarial growth. Inconsistent relationships were observed only between demographic variables (such as age, gender, and education) and measures of distress. However, individuals who showed adversarial growth over time were less likely to be distressed in the future than individuals who did not. Helgeson, Reynolds, and Tomich (2006) conducted a meta-analytic review of benefit finding and growth following traumatic experiences such as breast cancer, natural disasters, and rape. Results from 87 studies indicated that the effort of finding benefit amid adversity has several psychological consequences. Benefit finding reduced depression and increased positive well-being. On the other hand, individuals with higher levels of benefit finding also reported more intrusive and avoidant thoughts about the stressor. Helgeson et al. (2006) found that benefit finding was not related to anxiety, global distress, quality of life, or subjective reports of physical health. In general, the meta-analysis suggested that the effects of finding benefits are complex and dependent on various moderator variables, such as the amount of time that had passed since the stressor.

These results, while intriguing and important, should be viewed with some caution. Frazier et al. (2009) argued that the measure most commonly used in assessing posttraumatic growth, the Posttraumatic Growth Inventory (Tedeschi & Calhoun, 1996), is limited because it relies on retrospective reporting of events. Frazier et al. (2009) asked undergraduates to complete a series of measures tapping different aspects of personal growth and happiness. The change between pre- and posttest scores on these measures was assessed for respondents who reported a traumatic event between the two time periods. Frazier et al. (2009) found that pretest–posttest differences did not correlate well with the retrospective reports. Thus, issues of measurement need to be considered in examining these studies.

Posttraumatic Growth in Parents of Children With Disabilities

A small literature testifies to the potential for posttraumatic growth in parents of children with disabilities. One early study (Trute & Hauch, 1988) began with the assumption that much could be learned from families that had adapted well to the birth of a child with developmental disabilities. The researchers asked what kinds of factors led to positive adaptation in these families. Social workers selected families that displayed good adjustment, child emotional stability, and child developmental progress. The families were administered measures of family assessment and dyadic adjustment. Positive adaptation was not related to family income, nor was it related to the degree of the child's disability. However, two-parent families appeared to be at a distinct advantage over single-parent families, and successful families relied significantly on friends and family for emotional and social support. Trute and Hauch (1988) concluded that positive family functioning was related to the strength of the family system and its skillful utilization of family and friends.

Several studies have used qualitative analysis of interviews to identify themes in parental stories. Stainton and Besser (1998) interviewed six fathers and nine mothers regarding their views of the positive family impact, if any, of having a child with an intellectual disability. The researchers identified nine themes, including enhanced spirituality, increased tolerance and understanding, an increased sense of purpose, and a positive influence on others in their family and community. Stainton and Besser (1988) suggested that parents might have a view of their families that is different from that of the medical professionals serving their children, who tend to view the effects of disability on the family in purely negative terms. Similar themes have been found in several other qualitative studies (Kausar, Jevne, & Sobsey, 2003; Skinner, Bailey, Correa, & Rodriguez, 1999).

Scallan, Senior, and Reilly (2011) conducted a qualitative study of families of children with Williams syndrome. Williams syndrome is a genetic disorder caused by deletion of approximately 20 genes on chromosome 7. Individuals with Williams syndrome experience feeding difficulties, cardiovascular disease, growth abnormalities, and hypersensitivity to sound. In semistructured interviews with parents, Scallan et al. (2011) reported that 15 of 21 parents reported daily challenges associated with the tendency of individuals with Williams syndrome to be naïve and overly trusting of strangers. In addition, 18 of the parents rated their children's teachers as very poorly informed regarding how best to teach a child with Williams syndrome. At the same time, a majority of the parents agreed that their child brought joy to their family, had a positive impact on siblings, and changed their outlook on life.

In two studies with almost 500 children and young adults with developmental disabilities and their families, Blacher and Baker (2007) found that positive impact as measured by the Family Impact Questionnaire correlated negatively with behavior problems. Moreover, positive impact moderated the relationship between behavior problems and parental stress. The researchers also found that Latina mothers reported more positive family impact than Anglo mothers. Blacher and Baker (2007) suggested several possible explanations for this difference. One is that Latino families typically do not view their child as responsible for their behavior problems (Chavira, Lopez, Blacher, & Shapiro, 2000); as a consequence, parents are less likely to report negative emotions, such as anger and frustration, in relation to the child. Moreover, Blacher and Baker note that Latino families emphasize the embeddedness of the child in the family and take responsibility in their knowledge of their child. Thus, parents often feel that they are better able to make decisions regarding their child than the professionals who provide services. Latina mothers demonstrate a great deal of pride in their children and regard them in positive ways.

Hastings and Taunt (2002), in reviewing qualitative studies published to that date, identified 14 common themes that emerged in these studies. Common themes included a sense of accomplishment in having done one's best for the child, becoming a better person (e.g., less selfish), developing new skills, and increased spirituality. However, Hastings and Taunt (2002) noted some limitations of these studies. These themes did not derive from any particular theoretical orientation, nor did the studies directly test any particular hypotheses.

In addition to qualitative studies, some researchers have developed scales to measure positive experiences of parents of children with disabilities. Scorgie and Sobsey (2000) interviewed 15 parents of children with disabilities about their experiences as parents and then constructed a 59-item Life Management Survey from the interview themes. Responses to the survey indicated that parents strongly agreed that they had learned to speak out, had met new friends, and celebrated life more following the birth of their child with a disability. Hastings, Beck, and Hill (2005) examined the psychometric properties of the Positive Contributions Scale (PCS). The PCS is part of the Kansas Inventory of Parental Perceptions developed by Behr, Murphy, and Summers (cited in Hastings, Beck, & Hill, 2005). Hastings et al. (2005) asked 140 mothers and 60 fathers of children with intellectual disabilities to complete the PCS and related instruments. Both reliability and construct validity were satisfactory. Internal consistency was strong for all but one of the PCS subscales, and total PCS scores correlated positively with a scale that measured positive affect. Mothers generally reported more positive contributions than fathers. Mothers but not fathers experienced less parenting stress when they reported more positive experiences associated with raising their children with disabilities.

Kayfitz, Gragg, and Orr (2010) examined the relationship between positive experiences as measured by PCS and stress in parents of children with autism. Mothers reported significantly more positive experiences than fathers. Nonetheless, reports of positive experiences were negatively correlated with parenting stress for both mothers and fathers. Fathers' (but not mothers') reports of positive experiences were negatively associated with partners' reports of parenting stress. Although the causal nature of the relationship between positive impact and parental stress is not yet clear, such results suggest that encouraging parents to think of positive outcomes may help them enhance their relationships with their children.

There are both methodological and theoretical limitations to these studies. From a methodological standpoint, many of these studies lack a control group. Although it is promising to see transformational changes in parents of children with disabilities, the lack of a comparison group makes assessment of the extent to which the child's disability, some other life experiences, or both have contributed to the parent's growth problematic. In addition, several of the studies (Scorgie & Sobsey, 2000; Trute & Hauch, 1988) selected participants on the basis of overall satisfactory family adjustment, thus raising questions about the ability to generalize these results. Moreover, many of the studies were not theoretically grounded. Although it is possible to interpret these outcomes from the lens of positive psychology, most were not designed specifically to test or apply positive psychology principles.

An exception to the latter point is research based on Fredrickson's (1998) *broaden-and-build theory* of positive emotions. Fredrickson (1998) claimed that positive emotions—including joy, interest, contentment, pride, and love—broaden individuals' momentary thought–action repertoires, which in turn serves to build enduring physical, intellectual, social, and psychological resources. Research studies on the broaden-and-build model have found that positive emotions widen the scope of attention (Fredrickson & Branigan, 2005) and improve performance on certain cognitive tasks requiring attentional flexibility (Johnson, Waugh, & Fredrickson, 2010). Moreover, positive emotions contribute to resilience by helping individuals to "bounce back" from stressful experiences by undoing the cardiovascular effects of negative emotions (Fredrickson, Mancuso, Branigan, & Tugade, 2000).

Results of several recent studies suggest that the broaden-and-build framework may be applicable to parents of children with disabilities. Graungaard, Andersen, and Skov (2011) conducted a longitudinal, qualitative study of 11 parents of young children with severe disabilities. Their interviews focused on the question of why some parents coped better than others with the severe physical and emotional stress related to their child's disability. In particular, they examined how some parents created and maintained their energy and personal resources. Graungaard et al. found that some parents actively transformed both positive and negative experiences into resources through the use of positive reappraisal. For example, some parents transformed negative experiences into more optimistic reappraisals:

> We were told that he was not going to live very long and things like that all the time, so it has been up to us to have a hope . . . because otherwise . . . I can't live if I don't hope for something, I can't, even if maybe I know deep down that the hope is unrealistic. (p. 122[1])

Other examples of resource creation included parents who interpreted their child's progress in some area (e.g., fewer hospitalizations or seizures) as a hopeful sign for the future and parents who generated hope when meeting other parents of children with disabilities. The authors suggested that given the essential role that parent well-being plays in the care of the child, continued study of how parents create resources such as hope is needed.

---

[1]From "When Resources Get Sparse: A Longitudinal, Qualitative Study of Emotions, Coping and Resource-Creation When Parenting a Young Child With Severe Disabilities," by A. H. Graungaard, J. S. Andersen, and L. Skov, 2011, *Health, 15*, p. 122. Copyright 2011 by SAGE. Reprinted with permission.

Trute, Benzies, Worthington, Reddon, and Moore (2010) examined the effect of positive reappraisals on family functioning. A sample of 195 mothers of children with intellectual and developmental disabilities completed telephone interviews. The researchers found that 35% of the variance in family adjustment was accounted for by mothers' positive cognitive appraisal of family impacts of childhood disability and by their ratio of positive to negative affect. Trute et al. (2010) interpreted their results in light of Fredrickson et al.'s (2000) broaden-and-build model: Just as positive emotions may undo negative emotions, so positive appraisals may undo negative ones.

One other observation is relevant here. Although most of the studies pertaining to benefit finding in parents of children with developmental disabilities have focused on the emotional consequences for individual parents, how one parent appraises the family situation may influence the other parent. Recently, Samios, Pakenham, and Sofronoff (2012) have examined benefit finding and sense making in families of children with Asperger's syndrome from a family system perspective. Eighty-four couples completed measures of sense making (e.g., attributing a child with Asperger's syndrome to God's plan, seeing aspects of the syndrome in oneself), benefit finding (e.g., becoming more patient, becoming more aware of the problems faced by individuals with disabilities), and adjustment. Most interestingly, parents' sense making positively influenced not only their own adjustment but also that of their partners. The ways in which the processes of individual family members influence other members of the family are explored in greater detail in Chapter 4.

The upshot of this new wave of research on positive emotions in families of children with disabilities is reasonably clear. When investigators direct their attention to the positive changes that emerge in these families, some common themes appear and the presence of positive emotions and experiences facilitates family adjustment. Although there are remaining issues regarding how to assess and characterize these positive responses, they are an important if often neglected aspect of the lives of families of children with disabilities.

THE MIX OF EMOTIONS IN PARENTS

Let us take stock. We have seen that the experience of parenting a child with a developmental disability is a source of tremendous stress that can lead to adverse reactions including depressive symptoms in a significant minority of parents. At the same time, raising children with disabilities—perhaps because of their children's limitations in adapting to the world—may require parents to adapt and change in positive ways. Many of these parents see the struggles they have encountered as transformative.

These two lines of thought are not mutually exclusive. The experience of parents of children with disabilities is a mix of positive and negative emotions. A study by Kearney and Griffin (2001) brought out this aspect of the parenting experience. The parents they interviewed spoke of anguish and sorrow but also of hope, love, strength, and joy. These parents derived joy from their children, even as they drew sorrow from these same children. What emerges from this study and the survey of studies reviewed in this chapter is that the parents' experience of having a child with a developmental disability involves a mixture of emotions perhaps less often seen in parents of more typically developing children. The parenting experience is, in part, defined by the simultaneous presence of emotions often regarded as incompatible with one another. Perhaps this mix of emotions spurs parents on to the positive gains discussed in this chapter.

Green (2007) reinforced this point and added another. Green conducted a study of 81 mothers of children with developmental disabilities that included both quantitative and qualitative methods. Mothers completed measures of social stigma, caregiver burden, and benefits associated with caring for a disabled child. In addition, a subset of the mothers was interviewed, and Green identified several themes in these interviews. These mothers held positive views of their children and found benefits associated with raising a child with a disability. They strongly agreed with statements that they could see beneath people's appearances better than before and that their efforts were rewarded by the pride and joy they felt in their child's accomplishments.

Although these mothers also struggled with the challenge of caring for a disabled child on a 24/7 schedule, they did not perceive their burden as due to subjective emotional factors such as sadness. Rather, they associated it with more objective societal issues, including negative attitudes toward disabilities and inadequate support for those who care for children with disabilities. These mothers were burdened by the challenges of juggling work and family, securing medical care for their children, and financial issues rather than their own negative emotions. As the mothers put it, "we're tired, not sad" (Green, 2007, p. 150).

Green (2007) raises issues that I pursue in subsequent chapters. Social stigma is associated with disabilities, and parents experience challenges in working with medical and educational professionals. Before I discuss the larger social systems, however, we must better understand the family system—the interrelationships of roles and responsibilities within the family. I turn to the family system in Chapter 4.

4

FAMILY CHANGE AND REORGANIZATION

Well, it was sort of like there was a death in the family, really, because you sort of expect to have naturally good children. At first it was hard to accept, you know, to believe that it had happened to us . . . but once you accept it you're there for your daughter, you're there for your grandson. (Woodbridge, Buys, & Miller, 2011, p. 358)

Viewed as a system, the family is a group of individuals who play different and complementary roles. Some of the roles are internal to the home, including performance of tasks such as food preparation, house cleaning, and child care. Other roles serve to connect the family to the outside world through work, church, and community responsibilities. Traditionally, mothers were primarily responsible for childcare, while fathers did the work outside the home, but these roles have shifted significantly in recent decades and are now defined in different ways in different families. Nonetheless, all families need to find ways to allocate roles to their members.

Social roles are redefined when partners become parents. The introduction of a child into a family leads to both an increase in marital stability and, some scholars contend (McLanahan & Adams, 1987), a decline in marital quality (for a different view, see Galatzer-Levy, Mazursky, Mancini, & Bonanno, 2011). Parents must determine family and work roles

http://dx.doi.org/10.1037/14192-004
Families of Children With Developmental Disabilities: Understanding Stress and Opportunities for Growth,
by D. W. Carroll

and responsibilities. With multiple children, sibling relationships are added to the mix. Moreover, most families develop routines and rituals that are a common part of their everyday lives (Fiese et al., 2002). As children grow older and parents demand more of them in terms of household chores and schoolwork, their roles within the family shift. In addition, it is not uncommon for grandparents to live under the same roof, both performing various roles within the family and needing time and attention from parents.

All of these considerations apply to families of children with developmental disabilities, but they are more complex. Parents must balance the traditional parenting roles with work demands and the particular challenges of caring for a child with a disability, who might require frequent medical appointments, specialized equipment or services, and meetings with educational professionals. The sibling relationships are more complex as well; siblings try to learn how to play and function with one another, which may be especially challenging for a sibling of an older brother or sister with a disability.

In this chapter, I examine the family as a system. The first section deals with how parents adapt to their children with disabilities, the balance between family and work, and how roles between partners are arranged. I also discuss how the pattern of family adaptations influences marital quality. The second section deals with siblings, with an emphasis on the extent and causes of adjustment issues for young children with a brother or sister with a disability. The next section discusses grandparents and how their role may be redefined within the family. The final section discusses the contributions that routines and rituals make toward family resilience.

PARENTS

Patterns of Adaptation in Parent–Child Transactions

For many parents, raising a child with a disability requires flexibility in developing and adjusting parenting styles. Some parenting approaches that have been successful with typically developing children may not work as well with children with disabilities. A case in point is the *authoritative parenting style* advocated by Baumrind (1971). Baumrind found that a mixture of parental warmth, firm enforcement of rules, and reason was associated with greater independence and purposive behavior in preschool children. Woolfson and Grant (2006) studied parenting approaches and stress in parents of children with developmental disabilities and parents of typically developing children across younger (3–5 years) and older (9–11 years) age groups. Parents of typically developing children used more authoritative parenting with the older age group; however, the pattern was just the opposite for the families of children with disabilities. Woolfson and Grant suggested that the authoritative style was very stressful for parents of children with disabilities because of the amount of repetition needed and the limited success achieved. The time demands of authoritative parenting may also be a challenge for parents of children with disabilities due to other demands on parental time and energies. Woolfson and Grant suggested that parents of children with disabilities might choose to adopt a less demanding parenting style as a coping response to excessive demands as the child grows older.

Some children with disabilities have behavioral issues that pose significant challenges for their parents. They may include oppositional behavior, excessive anxiety, attentional issues, and difficulties with social competence (K. Crnic, Hoffman, Gaze, & Edelbrock, 2004). B. L. Baker, et al. (2003) discovered a transactional relationship between parenting stress and behavior problems: High levels of parenting stress contributed to worse child behavior over time, which in turn increased parenting stress. These relationships were similar for mothers and fathers.

Hastings and colleagues (Hastings, Daley, Burns, & Beck, 2006; Hastings & Lloyd, 2007) have examined expressed emotion in families of children with disabilities. *Expressed emotion* is a measure of the affective relationship between two individuals; high levels are characterized by criticism, hostility, and emotionally overinvolved attitudes. In a review of 11 studies, Hastings and Lloyd (2007) found evidence of high expressed emotion in some families with developmental disabilities. In addition, behavioral problems in children were related to parental expressed emotion. Thus, it appears that emotional overinvolvement may elicit inappropriate behavioral outcomes in children with disabilities.

Another form of adaptation is parental overprotection, which may be defined as a pattern of parenting that is appropriate for a child with a lower developmental level. Holmbeck et al. (2002; see also Vermaes, Gerris, & Janssens, 2007) examined observed and perceived parental overprotectiveness in families of children with spina bifida. Investigators studied 68 families with children with spina bifida (8–9 years of age) and a matched sample of 68 families with able-bodied children. Both questionnaire and observational measures indicated that mothers and fathers of children with spina bifida were significantly more overprotective than their counterparts in the able-bodied sample. This group difference was partially mediated by the children's cognitive ability. Mothers were more likely to be overprotective than fathers. Parental overprotectiveness was associated with less behavioral autonomy in children with spina bifida, which in turn was associated with more externalizing problems.

At the same time, there are examples of successful parental accommodation. Keogh, Garnier, Bernheimer, and Gallimore (2000) examined how families make both internal and external accommodations to children with developmental delays. Internal accommodations included changes in family organization in regard to domestic workload and childcare, whereas external accommodations referred to the use of outside resources such as social services or child peer groups. Chavira et al. (2000) examined the factors that may lead to successful and less successful family adaptations. Mothers who ascribed relatively lower responsibility to the child for behavioral issues were significantly less likely to report negative emotions (anger and frustration) and aggressive/harsh behavioral reactions than mothers who ascribed relatively high responsibility.

The nature of the accommodations that parents make may vary with the child's disability. Ly and Hodapp (2005) examined how parents of children with Williams syndrome and Prader–Willi syndrome interacted with their children as they worked on a puzzle task. Although both groups of children tend to have a lower level of cognitive functioning than typically developing age-mates, their intellectual profiles differ. In particular, children with Prader–Willi syndrome are relatively strong in visuospatial skills whereas children with Williams syndrome are weaker in this area. Although the children in the two groups were similar in their developmental levels (as measured by IQ tests), parents of children with Williams syndrome were more directive than parents of children with Prader–Willi syndrome. Ly and Hodapp suggested that parents responded to both the diagnosis and the particular behaviors that their children exhibited.

Sterling, Barnum, Skinner, Warren, and Fleming (2012) recently conducted a particularly interesting study of parental accommodations. Most studies that contrast syndromes employ between-subjects designs: They compare families and children with one syndrome with other families and children with another syndrome. This design has the limitation that the two groups of parents may differ on variables (e.g., socioeconomic status, family size) other than child disability. Sterling et al. employed a within-subject design, comparing the behavior of mothers when interacting with their child with a disability versus interacting with their child without a disability. In this study, the children had fragile X syndrome, a genetic disorder associated with intellectual disability, social anxiety, and repetitive behaviors. Sterling et al. found that although mothers used lots of praise and positive attention with both children, they used more behavior management techniques when interacting with their child with fragile X syndrome and adopted a more conversational style of interaction with the sibling.

Work–Family Balance

Most families with a child with a developmental disability have significant financial needs that require one or both parents to work outside the home. Young children with disabilities are significantly more likely to live in poverty than children without disabilities (S. L. Parish & Cloud, 2006). S. L. Parish and Cloud (2006) identified some of the contributing factors to this situation, including medical costs associated with children with disabilities along with the costs of childcare.

When parents work, there is often a "spillover effect" of work issues into the home. The juggling of work and family demands is particularly difficult for mothers. Shearn and Todd (2000) interviewed mothers of children with disabilities between 5 and 15 years old. The mothers found work to be difficult, and they encountered significant time demands and a lack of affordable childcare. In addition, the mothers found job opportunities were limited. Mothers who had part-time jobs often did low-status work for poor wages, with little opportunity to gain the skills needed for more attractive positions.

Other studies have found a tendency for mothers of children with disabilities to be limited to part-time employment because of childcare responsibilities. Lewis, Kagan, Heaton, and Cranshaw (1999) reported that parents of children with disabilities (ranging in age from 6 months to 29 years) enjoyed the same economic, psychological, and social benefits from participation in paid employment as did parents of children without disabilities. They concluded that the low levels of employment in mothers of children with disabilities were due to structural barriers, such as the lack of formal childcare. In support of this contention, Kagan, Lewis, Heaton, and Cranshaw (1999) found that when formal support mechanisms were in place, parents were able to combine work and caring roles more successfully. When the mechanisms were not in place, only the parents who could rely on family and friends to provide needed support were able to combine the roles. The authors suggested that increased workplace flexibility might provide the support that these mothers need.

Even as mothers of disabled children are frustrated by part-time employment, mothers in full-time positions often find the dual demands very stressful. Leiter, Krauss, Anderson, and Wells (2004) found that more than half of working mothers needed to reduce their work hours to care for their children with disabilities. In addition, more than half of the mothers at home full-time reported leaving paid employment due to their children's needs. Similarly, Witt, Gottlieb, Hampton, and Litzelman (2009) found that parents of children with new or ongoing health needs had more lost workdays than parents of children with fewer health care problems.

Workplace policies may ease parental burdens. One such policy is the Family Medical Leave Act, which provides medical leave for working parents when their children have medical needs. The working mothers interviewed by Jang and Appelbaum (2010) reported that although the Family Medical

Leave Act helped them take needed time off, it did not relieve financial concerns:

> Despite the flexibility, I experience stress. The clinic visits will be increasing and it is difficult to take off too much time because if I take time off from work to be with my son, for example if he is in the hospital, I can do it but I don't get paid. Or, if I need to take a week off to be with my son, I can still do it, but if I miss work I don't get paid. And if I am out too often, I lose my clients. (p. 325)

On the whole, Jang and Appelbaum concluded that parents in difficult situations can successfully develop strategies to achieve work–life balance and that workplace resources can assist them.

Balancing work and family responsibilities may be somewhat easier for mothers, particularly single mothers, once children are in school. Again, dual demands are more manageable when work and school schedules are flexible; even small workplace policies, such as the ability to call home to ensure that a child is home from school, can reduce role strain in mothers (Morris & Coley, 2004). These findings suggest that family-friendly policies, such as time off to attend to family needs, would reduce stress in working parents of children with disabilities.

In a recent study, Stein, Foran, and Cermak (2011) examined the application of a model of lifestyle balance to parents of children with autism spectrum disorder (ASD). The model identifies five dimensions: (a) rewarding and self-affirming relationships with others; (b) feeling interested, engaged, challenged, and competent; (c) creating meaning and a positive personal identity; (d) organizing time and energy to meet important personal goals and personal renewal; and (e) biological health and physical safety. They reviewed the research on parents of children with ASD in terms of the criteria and concluded that parents were less likely to achieve all of them successfully. The model would appear to have considerable utility in stimulating and integrating research on life–work balance for parents of children with disabilities.

Maternal and Paternal Roles and Well-Being

The stresses associated with juggling parenting and work do not fall evenly on mothers and fathers. Mothers bear a disproportionate burden of childcare responsibilities when one child has a developmental disability (Marcenko & Meyers, 1991). Bristol, Gallagher, and Schopler (1988) found that fathers of boys with disabilities assumed less responsibility than did comparison fathers for child care, even when the mother was employed. Moreover, decreased father involvement was specific to the disabled child, not to siblings, and was related to the severity of the child's atypical behaviors. Mothers in both disabled and comparison families reported more depressive symptoms and family disruptions than fathers.

Because women often have greater investment and responsibilities in childcare, it seems likely that child behavioral and health issues would influence maternal well-being more than paternal well-being. Research studies bear this out. Goldberg, Marcovitch, MacGregor, and Lojkasek (1986) found that fathers of developmentally delayed preschoolers reported fewer distress symptoms, more internal locus of control, higher self-esteem, and less support than mothers. Vermaes et al. (2007) reviewed studies of families of children with spina bifida and found that mothers were affected more negatively than fathers; mothers were also more likely to perceive dysfunction in the family roles.

There are indications that mothers and fathers are often influenced in different ways. In a study of parents of children with autism, Hastings (2003b) found that mothers and fathers showed similar levels of stress and depression. Nonetheless, they were affected by different variables. Maternal well-being was associated with both child behavior problems and their partner's mental health. In contrast, neither child behavior nor maternal mental health was associated with fathers' levels of stress. The impact of a child with disabilities on work is also different for mothers and fathers. Cuskelly, Pulman, and Hayes (1998) studied 20 families with a child with a disability and a comparison group of families without a child with a disability. Child disability had little effect on paternal employment but did influence maternal employment. Of the mothers of a child with a disability who were employed, all of them were employed part time, whereas only 50% of the mothers in the comparison group worked part time and the rest worked full time.

Marital Quality

Several studies have examined the interrelationships between marital quality and parenting stress in families of children with developmental disabilities. It appears that a bidirectional model is most appropriate here. There is evidence that the stress of parenting a disabled child may lessen marital intimacy (Fisman, Wolf, & Noh, 1989) and that marital stress may cause parent–child interactions to suffer (Floyd & Gallagher, 1997).

Kersh, Hedvat, Hauser-Cram, and Warfield (2006) found that greater marital quality predicted lower parenting stresses and fewer depressive symptoms for both mothers and fathers. In addition, marital quality predicted parenting efficacy for mothers, although not for fathers. Parenting self-efficacy, in turn, was related to child adjustment (Wanamaker & Glenwick, 1998).

Several studies suggest that there are relationships between paternal child involvement and marital quality. In a study of 243 Polish fathers,

Bragiel and Kaniok (2011) found that fathers' involvement in their child's life, care, rehabilitation, and education was positively correlated with marital satisfaction of fathers. Father involvement is also important for mothers: Simmerman, Blacher, and Baker (2001) examined both parents' perceptions of father involvement with a young child with a disability. Most mothers reported that they were satisfied with the extent of fathers' help. One intriguing finding was that marital adjustment was more strongly correlated with maternal satisfaction with father involvement with the child than the actual extent of paternal involvement.

Other studies have explored whether divorce rates differ for couples with a child with a disability relative to those with healthy children. The largest study (Witt, Riley, & Coiro, 2003) compared divorce rates in 5,089 families of children with disabilities and more than 24,000 families of children without disabilities. The prevalence of divorce was somewhat higher in the disability group (14.3%) than the nondisability group (11.4%). In their meta-analysis of marital adjustment in parents of children with disabilities, Risdal and Singer (2004) examined six studies that compared the prevalence of divorce in families of children with and without disabilities. All of the studies found higher percentages of divorce in the disability group, but the differences were typically small: The effect sizes ranged from .09 (in the Witt et al., 2003, study) to .38, with a weighted average of .21. Thus, divorce rates were higher when there is a child with a disability, but only slightly. Risdal and Singer (2004) concluded that the effect is smaller than many investigators might have predicted.

A more recent study provided an important qualification. Hatton, Emerson, Graham, Blacher, and Llewellyn (2010) found that children with early cognitive delay were more likely than children without delays to be born into a household without both biological parents. That is, the difference in the percentage of homes with two biological parents preceded the child's birth and subsequent discovery of cognitive delay. This result raised questions regarding whether the stress associated with parenting a child with a disability is the principal cause of separation or divorce in families and suggested that broader socioeconomic factors must be considered.

SIBLINGS

Being a sibling of a child with a developmental disability often leads to a complex array of emotions. Children may resent the amount of parental time and attention their sibling receives and the caregiving responsibilities they may have to undertake to assist in the care of their sibling. Nonetheless, siblings may also appreciate that the sibling has special needs. As a result, resentment or even overt hostility is often more likely to be directed at parents than siblings.

Siblings of children with some disabilities may have their own genetic risk. For example, siblings of individuals with ASD carry the risk of the broader autism phenotype, in which individuals have some of the characteristics associated with autism although typically at a reduced level. Thus, siblings may experience learning problems, adjustment difficulties, and other issues not because of their experience with their siblings but because of their own genetic susceptibility.

Several studies have reported adjustment problems in children with disabled siblings. In an early study, McHale and Gamble (1989) studied children with and without siblings with intellectual disabilities. In all cases, the child with a disability was the younger sibling. The authors used home interviews of mothers and children. Children completed measures of self-esteem, depression, and anxiety and also rated their interactions with their disabled siblings. Compared with children with typically developing siblings, children with siblings with disabilities reported spending more time in caregiving activities and more favorable perceptions of how well the siblings got along. They also reported that negative interactions with their mothers were more frequent. Children with siblings with disabilities, particularly girls, also reported poorer adjustment on anxiety and depression measures. These children tended to have higher scores on measures of anxiety and depression, yet nearly all of the scores fell within the normal range. Although the study provided evidence of adjustment problems for children with younger disabled siblings, the problems were comparatively mild.

Sibling perception of differential parental treatment contributes to adjustment issues. McHale and Gamble (1989) found that children's satisfaction with how their parents treated them relative to their siblings was negatively correlated with sibling depression and anxiety. That is, children who were satisfied that their younger siblings needed additional time from their parents were less anxious or depressed. McHale and Pawletko (1992) explored some of the contradictory or ambivalent emotional reactions that siblings may experience. They found that typically developing siblings felt guilty when they received more favorable treatment from their parents. Moreover, McHale and Pawletko found that older children felt left out or neglected even if they believed that their parents' attention to younger or disabled siblings was legitimate.

Sibling relationships may vary with the type of disability. Petalas, Hastings, Nash, Lloyd, and Dowey (2009) compared siblings of children with intellectual disabilities with and without autism. Mothers rated the emotional adjustment of siblings. Siblings of children with both intellectual disabilities and autism had more emotional problems compared with siblings of children with intellectual disabilities alone or normative data. Thus, the presence of autism appears to increase the emotional problems of siblings over and above the presence of intellectual disabilities. Similarly, Fisman, Wolf, Ellison, and Freeman (2000) found that siblings of children with pervasive developmental disorder showed significantly more adjustment problems compared with siblings of children with Down syndrome and with control children.

As with parents, child behavior problems are a significant factor in sibling responses. Neece, Blacher, and Baker (2010) found that child behavior problems played a significant role in how children were influenced by siblings with intellectual disabilities. In the Neece et al. study, children with autism were excluded. Mothers and fathers reported siblings to be more negatively influenced than were siblings of typically developing children. However, when child behavior problems were accounted for, there was no longer a significant relationship between child intellectual status and the impact on siblings.

Other studies point to the difficulties in developing a relationship with a sibling with autism. Kaminsky and Dewey (2001) examined sibling relationships of children with autism or Down syndrome and typically developing children. Sibling relationships in families of children with autism were associated with less intimacy than the two comparison groups. At the same time, both siblings of children with autism and siblings of children with Down syndrome expressed greater admiration for and less competition with their siblings than did siblings of typically developing children. Mulroy, Robertson, Aiberti, Leonard, and Bower (2008) assessed parent perceptions of siblings of children with Down syndrome or Rett syndrome. Parents identified both benefits and disadvantages. Although parents expressed concerns about time constraints and the difficulties in forming relationships between siblings, they also acknowledged that siblings displayed more compassion and patience.

One might surmise that birth order matters here. After all, if a child is born after a sibling with a disability, family adaptation to disability issues might be well under way and the younger child might tacitly understand that "this is the way it is done in our family." Some younger siblings may only belatedly realize that not every child has an older brother or sister with a disability. In contrast, if the disabled child were the younger sibling, it would seem that the possibilities of resentment on the part of the older sibling are greater. Not only has the older child lost the full attention of his or her parents, but also the younger sibling with the special needs now commands a disproportionate amount of that attention. Although such speculations may be reasonable, scant data are available on the issue, and what does exist does not support these conjectures (Levy-Wasser & Katz, 2004).

Sibling adjustment contributes to overall family and marital functioning. Rivers and Stoneman (2003) found a relationship between marital stress and the quality of sibling relationships when one child had autism. When the level of marital stress was greater, sibling relationships were more compromised. Similar results have been reported for siblings of children with pervasive developmental disorder, Down syndrome, and spina bifida (Bellin & Rice, 2009; Fisman et al., 2000). These correlational findings leave open the question of the nature of the causal link between marital stress and sibling relationships.

Although some studies find adjustment problems in siblings, others have found that siblings adjust quite well to their nonnormative family experience. A meta-analysis (Rossiter & Sharpe, 2001) found a small negative effect of having a sibling with a developmental disability but that some studies have also found positive consequences for siblings. Siblings, particularly older siblings and girls, often assume a greater role in caregiving toward their disabled sibling (Cuskelly & Gunn, 2003; Hannah & Midlarsky, 2005). This role is associated with greater empathy in siblings (Cuskelly & Gunn, 2003) and may encourage the greater compassion and understanding of individuals with disabilities that parents report (Mulroy et al., 2008).

However, parents and children may view the role of a sibling somewhat differently. Barak-Levy, Goldstein, and Weinstock (2010) studied siblings of children with autism. Although superficially these siblings appeared to be doing well (e.g., absence of high levels of behavioral problems), the investigators suggested that a deeper analysis revealed some psychological issues. These children had a much lower level of participation in child activities and poorer social relations and school performance. The siblings saw themselves as responsible for considerably higher levels of assistance within the home than their peers. Whereas parents regarded the helping behavior as a positive, the children viewed the additional burden with some distress. Thus, the caregiving role presents both challenges and opportunities. It may enable siblings to develop prosocial behaviors and empathy while limiting their ability to engage socially with their peers or engage in school and extracurricular activities. Some siblings may come to view their responsibilities as a burden, thus leading to adjustment problems.

Sibling adjustment issues may be minimized by social support. Wolf, Fisman, Ellison, and Freeman (1998) found that social support received from parents, teachers, and close friends was negatively correlated with externalizing behavior problems. The effectiveness of social support appeared to be greater in children with siblings with pervasive developmental disorder than in children with siblings with Down syndrome. Hastings (2003a) found similar results in children with siblings with autism. Siblings in families with a less severely autistic child had fewer adjustment problems when more formal social support (in-home behavioral intervention) was also available in the family. Studies of social support are discussed more fully in Chapter 7.

In sum, sibling adjustment is complex and multifaceted. In the discussion of stress in Chapter 3, it was observed that although parenting a child with a disability is a tremendously stressful challenge, some parents emerge from the experience with considerable personal growth. Less attention has been paid to the potential positive consequences for siblings. In part, this may be due to a general tendency for scholars and society to view disability primarily in negative terms. However, young children may not be fully prepared to appreciate the positive outcomes associated with having a sibling with a developmental disability. As children grow into adulthood, the way in which they think about their brother or sister may change. Some siblings become protective, for example correcting classmates who use inappropriate language, and many siblings eventually adopt a position of advocacy at some point in their lives. Our discussion of how sibling relationships change over the years continues in Chapter 8.

GRANDPARENTS

Just as parents of children with disabilities must adapt to unexpected roles, grandparents may find themselves in an unfamiliar and challenging position. The implicit assumption for many grandparents, particularly grandmothers, is that they will serve as educational experts for their children, offering advice on matters from toilet training to discipline. As young adults become parents, they may come to appreciate their own mothers more, and their mothers may reciprocate by acknowledging their adult children's newfound status as parents. Many grandparents look forward to this period of their life, one in which their knowledge is appreciated and valued while the demands on their time are limited.

When a child has a developmental disability, these expectations are largely put aside, and the primary role of the grandparent is to support his or her adult children in their time of need. However, as Simons (1987) observed, grandparents may feel a double grief. They may grieve the loss of the grandchild they anticipated and experience a deep sadness at their own adult children's pain. The latter grief may render the grandparents unable to provide the support their children need at a critical time of their lives. Thus, the diagnosis of a grandchild with a disability is a significant emotional experience for grandparents.

Woodbridge, Buys, and Miller (2009) conducted a qualitative study of 22 Australian grandparents whose grandchild had been diagnosed with a disability. These grandparents reported a prolonged sense of sadness pertaining to both their grandchild and their child: "There is just a sadness you carry with you all the time. There is a double grief because you grieve for the child but you also grieve for your child" (p. 39). Other respondents described the experience in terms of grief at the loss of the grandchild they had expected.

On the other hand, these grandparents also felt a sense of pride in their family's ability to adapt to unexpected challenges.

In a review of the literature, Hastings (1997) reported that grandparents served as a source of both support and conflict for parents. The initial responses of grandparents included shock, denial, and depression, but over time grandparents came to fulfill a number of supportive functions in the family, providing both instrumental support (e.g., grocery shopping, babysitting) and emotional support (e.g., encouragement, listening). At the same time, grandparents sometimes constituted an additional source of stress for parents. Parents needed to provide emotional support for grandparents mourning the loss of a "normal" grandchild and often disagreed with grandparents on issues related to the child's developmental progress. In particular, grandparents were more likely to believe that there was nothing wrong with the child, a finding reported by other investigators (D. Gray, 2002) at a time when parents were struggling with obtaining needed services for their children.

Gender roles influence these relationships. Hastings, Thomas, and Delwiche (2002) found that grandparent support and conflict were associated with mothers' but not fathers' ratings of stress associated with parenting a child with Down syndrome. Trute, Worthington, and Hiebert-Murphy (2008) found similar results in families of children with ASD, cerebral palsy, fragile X syndrome, and Down syndrome. Grandmother support was an important predictor of maternal stress but not paternal stress.

S. Katz and Kessel (2002) explored the perceptions and beliefs of grandparents regarding their grandchild with a developmental disability. The researchers noted a discrepancy between the grandparents' positive attitudes and overt acceptance of their own grandchildren and their negative attitudes toward children with disabilities in general. Grandparents were also ambivalent about the value of intervention with children with disabilities; they hoped that intervention services would help the children but often doubted that it would. Parents determined the degree of involvement of grandparents with their grandchildren, sometimes excluding the grandparents. One grandmother commented:

> My daughter-in-law never allowed me to feed the child as a baby. She did not think that I could do it right. She is very protective of the child. . . . If we were to wait for them to invite us to come we would never get there. Today we feel closer, there is more mutual trust and respect. . . . I have learnt that if I want to help the child, I have to do everything through my daughter-in-law, letting her decide. (S. Katz & Kessel, 2002, p. 123)

Greater cooperation between grandparents and their adult children occurred when grandparents were perceived as supportive and nonjudgmental. Moreover, involvement with the grandchild tended to strengthen the grandparents' relationship with the adult child. As noted by other researchers, grandmothers tended to be more involved than grandfathers.

Hillman (2007) offered several policy recommendations with particular attention to grandparents of children with autism. Grandparents need accurate information about the symptoms and treatments for autism and need to develop concrete skills, including technology skills, for successfully interacting with their grandchildren with autism. Hillman suggested that support groups might be useful for some grandparents. In addition, some grandparents may wish to become involved in advocacy efforts to support their children and grandchildren in, for example, obtaining needed educational services. Overall, grandparents may need help in redefining their role within the family.

ROUTINES, RITUALS, AND RESILIENCE

As noted at the outset of this chapter, routines and rituals can help provide a sense of order in a family. Fiese et al. (2002) distinguished between *family routines* and *family rituals*. Routines are observable practices, whereas family rituals are symbolic representations of collective events. For example, a mealtime routine may involve instrumental communication regarding who should pick up milk on the way home from work, whereas a mealtime ritual may include conversations that establish family values. Fiese and colleagues found that both routines and rituals were related to parenting competence, child adjustment, and marital satisfaction.

Although it is more difficult to establish routines and rituals in families with children with developmental disabilities, such practices may be especially valuable for these families. For families under considerable stress, routines and rituals may provide a much-needed element of order and predictability. Spagnola and Fiese (2007) examined rituals in families of children with disabilities from the perspective of the transactional model in which parents and children both influence each other and evolve over time. For example, a child born with a congenital heart condition raises parental concerns about the child waking during the night, leading parents to provide a soft back rub to the child before bed, followed by the child sleeping through the night and the parent developing a sense of confidence. Moreover, children with disabilities often receive early intervention in the home, and it is possible to embed early interventions within existing family routines.

Several studies have examined the efforts of parents of children with disabilities to establish rituals and routines. Rehm and Bradley (2005) conducted a qualitative study of families of children who were medically fragile, technology-dependent, or developmentally delayed. The parents encouraged behaviors and family routines that promoted a sense of normalcy, even if it was a different type of normalcy than that experienced by other families. Parents appreciated when their child could attend school on a regular basis because it provided an opportunity for the child to participate in a normal part of childhood. Regular school attendance also granted parents a respite from childcare, thus permitting them to attend to other family chores and errands. Similarly, parents chose leisure activities in light of their child's needs. When families had children who required extra supplies and machinery, they often chose to take trips by car, or simply stayed home.

The establishment of routines and rituals appears to promote family resilience. Knestricht and Kuchey (2009) studied 20 families of children with special needs in an effort to determine what factors were most predictive of family resilience. They found that family routines, such as a structured system for doing the laundry for a family of six children, were common in resilient families. In addition, these families tended to include their children with disabilities in family activities to the extent possible, rather than deprive themselves of these activities in light of the child's disability. Similarly, Heiman (2002), in a study discussed in the previous chapter, found that parents of children with an intellectual, physical, or learning disability tried to maintain routines in their lives, for example by drawing upon the support of extended family members to help with child care. Although these reports are preliminary and impressionistic, they suggest that the effort to develop predictability may promote resilience in families of children with disabilities.

In summary, when parents have a child with a disability, a central task is to determine how to allocate family time and resources to provide care for the child while maintaining the functioning of the entire family (Guralnick, 2004). Guralnick suggested that parents respond to these tasks by investing resources into various domains, including the domestic workload, marital roles, health services, and child care. This chapter has examined how parents invest in the family system by reorganizing roles, adapting interactions, attending to the needs of siblings and grandparents, and developing routines and rituals. Parents must balance tasks that maintain the functioning and health of the family system with those that involve the interaction of the family with other social systems. Two of the most important systems are the medical and educational contexts that provide services for children with disabilities. In the next chapter, I examine the medical context.

5

MEDICAL ISSUES AND MEDICAL PROFESSIONALS

But it would be easier if we had cooperation with the professionals, instead of this fight to get their attention . . . to try to break through the shell of professionalism. It is like: I am the expert and you are the ones who don't know anything . . . (Graungaard & Skov, 2007, p. 304).

Children with developmental disabilities often have significant health care needs. Individuals with Down syndrome frequently have heart issues, and those with spina bifida may require the use of a wheelchair. Many children with cerebral palsy need assistive technology to communicate effectively. Other children, such as those ultimately diagnosed with autism spectrum disorder (ASD) or pervasive developmental disorder, may require many medical appointments before an accurate diagnosis can be made. Many children with developmental disabilities require prescription medications, frequent visits to physicians and therapists, and intermittent hospitalizations.

Managing the medical issues of children with disabilities can be emotionally and physically draining for parents. Medical visits are time-consuming and expensive, and parents need to become familiar with insurance reimbursement and other means of paying for medical appointments,

http://dx.doi.org/10.1037/14192-005
Families of Children With Developmental Disabilities: Understanding Stress and Opportunities for Growth,
by D. W. Carroll

equipment, and medications. Parents need to do all of this while handling the variety of other tasks already described—attending to other family members, balancing family and work, assigning different family roles, and so forth.

In this chapter, I examine how parents deal with the complex medical challenges associated with having a child with significant health care needs. The first section discusses how families gain access to medical care and examines parent satisfaction with medical care. The second section deals with communication issues between medical providers and parents and the impact communication has on medical care for children with disabilities.

GAINING ACCESS TO MEDICAL CARE

Prevalence of Children With Special Health Needs

Let us begin by considering the scope of the problem. The most detailed recent estimates come from the National Survey of Children with Special Health Care Needs (NS-CSHCN). The survey employed the definition developed by the Maternal and Child Health Bureau that states that a child with a special health care need (a) has or is at risk for having a physical, developmental, behavioral, or emotional condition and (b) requires health or related services of a type or amount beyond that required by children generally (McPherson et al., 1998). Kogan, Strickland, and Newacheck (2009), using the 2001 NS-CSHCN data, estimated that one of every seven children younger than 18 years in the United States (10.2 million) can be classified as having special health care needs. These data included some conditions, such as childhood diabetes, that fall outside conventional definitions of developmental disability. Ultimately, the percentage of children with developmental disabilities depends on the strictness of the definition. Boyle, Decoufle, and Yeargin-Allsopp (1994) estimated that 17% of children in the United States have or ever had a developmental disability. In this study, disabilities included emotional or behavioral problems, learning disabilities, delays in growth and development, seizure disorders, and sensory deficits.

Children with disabilities, however defined, require a disproportionately large percentage of health care resources. Newacheck, Inkelas, and Kim (2004) compared the utilization of medical services in children with and without disabilities. Children with disabilities utilized many more services than did children without disabilities. The largest differences were for hospital days (464 vs. 55 days per 1,000), visits to health professionals other than physicians (3.0 vs. 0.6), and home health provider days (3.8 vs. 0.04).

Gaining Access to the Medical Home

Another central issue for many parents of children with disabilities is how to receive coordinated medical care. Children with disabilities often have complex medical issues that require the attention of several medical specialists. At the least, scheduling and bringing their children to multiple appointments on separate days can be a hassle for parents. In addition, parents often need to take time off from work for these office visits. Worse, when many different specialists are providing services, issues concerning communication between providers may arise, which complicates the coordination of medical care.

The American Academy of Pediatrics, recognizing this problem, developed a policy statement regarding care for children with special health care needs (American Academy of Pediatrics, 2002). The policy asserted that the medical care of infants, children, and adolescents with special needs should be comprehensive, coordinated, and family-centered. The statement also defined the concept of a *medical home,* an environment in which a well-trained physician provides primary care and helps to manage and facilitate virtually all aspects of pediatric care. The policy statement identifies 10 characteristics of a medical home, including family-centered services (e.g., a partnership with families based on trust and respect for family diversity), coordination of care (e.g., the family, the physician, and other service providers work as an organized team to implement a care plan), and interaction with early intervention programs (e.g., childhood education and child care programs that need to be aware of a child's health needs).

Strickland et al. (2004) examined parent perceptions regarding access to a medical home. They selected five components of a medical home: (a) a usual place for care, (b) a personal physician or nurse, (c) no difficulty in obtaining needed referrals, (d) needed care coordination, and (e) family-centered care received. Results of the survey indicated that approximately half of children with special health care needs receive care that meets all five criteria. Almost 90% of the parents reported having a personal doctor or nurse, and roughly two thirds reported receiving family-centered services. However, coordination between medical professionals is a common problem: Less than 40% of parents reported receiving effective care coordination.

Financial Barriers to Health Care Access

Several studies have documented the financial barriers for gaining health care services and equipment for children with special health care needs. Newacheck and Kim (2005) provided nationally representative data on total health care expenses, out-of-pocket health care expenses, and the extent to which out-of-pocket expenses are financially burdensome for families. Compared with children without special health care needs, children with special health care needs had three times higher health care expenditures. Medical insurance provided good coverage of inpatient hospital care but poor coverage of dental care expenses. Families of children with special health care needs experiencing high out-of-pocket expenses (exceeding 5% of family income) were approximately 11 times more likely to be from households with incomes below 200% of the federal poverty level. Overall, families caring for children with health issues have much higher expenditures, including out-of-pocket expenditures, than families of healthy children. Health insurance provides important yet incomplete protection.

Nolan, Orlando, and Liptak (2007) compared access to medical services and medical equipment. They reported that most families had few problems accessing acute care or therapy services such as physical or occupational therapy, especially with the help of their providers. However, 46% reported some difficulty getting needed medical equipment. Parents also ranked their concerns related to medical care for their children. They ranked access to acute medical care as their primary concern, involvement in decision making as second, and communication with professionals as third.

Newacheck, Hughes, Hung, Wong, and Stoddard (2000) estimated that 7.3% of children (4.7 million) in the United States experienced at least one unmet health care need. Dental care was the most prevalent unmet need. Poor or near-poor children were about three times more likely to have an unmet need. Van Dyck, Kogan, McPherson, Weissman, and Newacheck (2004) found that a substantial minority of children with special health care needs (17.7%) experienced unmet health needs or lacked critical elements of family-centered health care (33.5%). These researchers also documented the impact on families: 20.9% reported that the child's health care caused financial problems and 29.9% reported cutting back or quitting work because of the child's condition. Adams, Newacheck, Park, Brindis, and Irwin (2007) documented that the lack of insurance was a greater problem for individuals after age 18. The disappearance of this social safety net represents a significant stressor for parents as their children with developmental disabilities approach young adulthood.

Disparities in access to health care among ethnic and racial groups result from financial issues and cultural attitudes. Blumberg, Read, Avila, and Bethell (2010) found that Hispanic children from Spanish-speaking households were only one third as likely to be identified as CSHCN than were other Hispanic and non-Hispanic White families. In addition, Spanish-speaking families had a higher prevalence of several developmentally related conditions. Javier, Huffman, Mendoza, and Wise (2010) found that children with special health care needs from immigrant families were more likely to be uninsured, lacked a usual source of care, had delays in health care, and had had no visits to the doctor in the past year. Moreover, the quality of health care received is an issue. Magaña, Parish, Rose, Timberlake, and Swaine (2012) found that Black and Latino children had poorer quality of health care in five of six indicators (e.g., having a personal doctor or nurse) than did White children. In addition, cultural attitudes may interfere with families' access to health care. D. L. Baker, Miller, Dang, Yaangh, and Hansen (2010) found that Southeast Asian families (Hmong and Mien) perceived that reliance on government programs was not appropriate. This attitude interfered with community acceptance and use of available services.

Parent Satisfaction With Family-Centered Services

As noted above, family-centered services are considered an integral part of the medical home for a child with special health care needs. S. King, Teplicky, King, and Rosenbaum (2004) reviewed the literature on the efficacy of family-centered services, which they defined as follows:

> Family-centered service is made up of a set of values, attitudes, and approaches to services for children with special needs and their families. Family-centered service recognizes that each family is unique; that the family is the constant in the child's life; and that they are the experts on the child's abilities and needs. The family works together with service providers to make informed decisions about the services and supports the child and family receive. In family-centered service, the strengths and needs of all family members are considered. (p. 79)

S. King et al. regarded family-centered service as a holistic approach to intervention analogous to Carl Rogers's client-centered therapy. The three aspects of caregiving that are common in this service are information exchange, respectful and supportive care, and partnership or enabling.

Research indicates that family-centered services lead to positive outcomes for both the child and the family members. G. King, King, Rosenbaum, and Goffin (1999) surveyed 164 parents of children with cerebral palsy, spina bifida, or hydrocephalus. They found that family-centered services led to a small but significant reduction in parental stress and were a significant predictor of parents' well-being. Parents were appreciative of the attention given by their medical providers to social support, child behavior problems, and family functioning. Law et al. (2003) examined factors affecting parents' perception of service delivery for children with disabilities. The authors found that the strongest predictor of parent satisfaction was the parents' perception of the extent to which service practices were family-centered. In particular, parents were more satisfied when there were fewer places where services were received.

Dempsey and Keen (2008) provide the most recent review of studies on the effectiveness of family-centered services. Although they acknowledged a growing body of evidence that documented the efficacy of the approach, they also pointed out that the results are complex and that much is not known. They reviewed 35 studies conducted since 1987 and found evidence that family-centered programs improved parental locus of control and self-efficacy. Although the evidence was not conclusive, several studies suggested an association between parental control attributions and parent stress and well-being. They also noted that it is crucial for the field to undertake longitudinal studies to permit more confident assertions about the causal relationships between variables and the need for further research into the extent to which these programs influence child development and reduce child behavior problems. Given that most current research is cross-sectional, it is not possible to conclude that family-centered programs improve child and family outcomes over time.

COMMUNICATING WITH MEDICAL PROFESSIONALS

For parents of children with special medical needs, an effective relationship with medical professionals such as physicians, nurses, and physical therapists is essential in making informed decisions about the child's medical care. Effective relationships with medical professionals depend on successful communication that, in turn, rests on an appreciation of the respective roles of patient and physician in our society. In this section, I begin with some sociological insights into the nature of the roles of physician and patient in society. Then I examine how these roles shape medical visits.

Sociological Considerations

Parsons (1951, 1975) argued that medical practices rest on an asymmetrical relationship between patient and physician. Physicians are regarded as experts to whom patients go for highly specialized knowledge about medical conditions. Patients provide data to physicians regarding their symptoms, and physicians draw on their knowledge to provide a diagnosis for the patient's problem. The diagnosis not only provides the basis for the management of the condition but also grants the patient access to what Parsons referred to as "the sick role." This role shapes the medical encounter. Thus, an examination of the nature of physician–patient communication is worthwhile, with particular interest in the communication of diagnoses.

There has been considerable study of medical communication—primarily conversations between physicians and patients—over the past few decades.

This includes reviews of the methodology of conversation analysis (Heritage, 2005; Wooffitt, 2005) and its application to medical communication (Heritage & Maynard, 2006; Perakyla, 1997). I begin by examining discourse between physicians and patients and then turn to conversations between physicians and parents and conversations between physicians, parents, and children. Finally, I consider the impact of the discussions on families of children with disabilities.

Communication Between Physicians and Patients

The setting in which physicians and patients converse has been referred to as an institutional setting to distinguish it from personal settings (Clark, 1996). In *personal settings*, two or more participants engage in a free exchange of conversational turns. In *institutional settings*, the speech exchanges resemble ordinary conversation but are constrained by institutional rules. In particular, the conversation is not between equals. In institutional discourse, one participant (for example, a judge, teacher, or therapist) is generally considered the expert.

I begin by considering an admittedly simplistic model of what physicians do during a medical visit. First, the physician takes the patient's history and listens carefully as the patient reports symptoms and concerns. In essence, the patient is the expert on these symptoms. Second, the physician interprets the patient's reports and suggests a diagnosis. Third, the physician suggests a course of action (e.g., medical test, medication). These tasks are not necessarily organized sequentially; office visits may interweave data, interpretation, and suggestion in a complex pattern. Nonetheless, physicians undertake each of these tasks. Conversation analysis has focused primarily on the diagnostic part of the office visit: how and in what way the physician communicates the diagnosis of the condition to the patient. Heath (1992) has observed that the diagnosis is a pivotal point in the consultation between patient and physician. It marks the conclusion of the "data-gathering" phase and begins (and in fact is the basis for) the discussion of possible treatments. As Parsons (1951, 1975) suggested, it is the province of the physician to form this medical judgment.

Research reveals that physicians often spend more time identifying symptoms and recommending treatment options than in discussing diagnoses. In an early study, Byrne and Long (1976) observed that physicians often moved quickly from conducting a physical examination to recommending a course of treatment without much discussion or justification of why they had made a particular diagnosis. Byrne and Long (1976) suggested that the power asymmetry between patient and physician might be one reason why diagnoses are discussed so briefly. However, patients also contribute to the brevity of the diagnostic segment. Heath (1992) observed that patients are often reticent to respond immediately after a diagnosis is made; the physician often waits briefly, and then proceeds to discuss treatments. The relative absence of patient response may be partly attributable to the factual manner in which diagnoses are often presented to patients. When physicians present their diagnoses in the form of a question or with some tentative language (*I think . . .*), patients are more likely to discuss the diagnosis as opposed to when they simply announce the diagnosis (Heath, 1992).

Communication Between Physicians and Parents

Some of the earliest conversations between parents and medical professionals occur in the context of diagnosis. As we saw in Chapter 2, the experience of parents varies significantly with the nature of the child's disability. Parents of children with Down syndrome are typically informed very early in a child's life, whereas the wait is much longer for parents of children with ASD. Some studies have moved beyond the question of when the diagnosis is delivered to examine how physicians deliver diagnostic news.

Empirical studies of medical communication of diagnoses indicate that physicians proceed cautiously when presenting diagnostic labels to parents. Using videotapes of informing interviews involving clinicians and parents, V. T. Gill and Maynard (1995) found that physicians used conversational techniques that enable parent responses to enter into the news delivery and labeling process. Maynard (2004) explored the distinction between "citing the evidence" and "asserting the condition" in conversations between parents and physicians. In the former case, physicians present information in the form of tests that may lead the parent to suspect possible conditions, but the physician does not actually assert or identify the condition. Clinicians often delay asserting the condition, which can be more confrontational and presumptive. They may postpone difficult discussions by citing the evidence prior to asserting the condition.

Similar themes emerged in a study by Abrams and Goodman (1998) that discussed how parents and professionals negotiate bad news in diagnostic situations. Participants included parents of children (mean age, 37.7 months) suspected of developmental delays and several types of professionals (psychologists, social workers, and pediatricians). Professionals shied away from explicit use of diagnostic labels, preferring instead to use rate descriptors (e.g., *slow*). Professionals and parents made both optimistic and pessimistic statements. The professionals showed considerable sensitivity to parental statements. When parents showed despair, professionals held out hope; when parents were unrealistic, professionals made more blunt statements. The authors suggested that the vagueness of some physicians leaves a large contested area in which parties may make claims and counterclaims. Although much of the literature has focused on the power differential between parents and professionals, Abrams and Goodman found that parents and professionals jointly construct diagnoses of developmental disabilities.

Skotko, Capone, and Kishnani (2009) reviewed empirical studies to identify best practices in delivering Down syndrome diagnoses. Based on parental reactions, they concluded that mothers preferred to learn the news from a physician (even though nurses, medical residents, and others often delivered such diagnoses) as soon as possible and in a private setting. Parents preferred the information presented to be accurate, balanced, and limited to the most immediate medical issues. Moreover, parents often remember the first words physician used in this context: Parents preferred to first be congratulated on the birth of their infant, rather than experience a conversation that begins with condolences.

Parent preferences diverge somewhat from those of medical professionals. Sheets, Best, Brasington, and Will (2011) presented 993 parents of children with Down syndrome and 389 genetic counselors with a list of 100 items that could be discussed during genetic counseling and asked them to judge whether each of the items was essential, important, or not too important for inclusion in the first discussion of the diagnosis. Some commonalities were observed: Both groups thought that information about early intervention centers and local support groups was essential.

The results also indicated that some items of information were valued differently in the two groups. Genetic counselors believed that an explanation of the diagnosis by chromosome analysis and the possibility that the child might need heart surgery were essential. In contrast, parents valued information about the abilities and potential of individuals with Down syndrome more than clinical details. They valued knowing that children with Down syndrome were more like other children than different from them. They also placed greater value in having contact with a family that was raising a child with Down syndrome. The information from this study should provide guidance for health care professionals interested in providing balanced information about Down syndrome to new parents.

Communication Between Physicians, Parents, and Children

When parents bring their children to see a pediatrician, the parents typically speak for their children. This is particularly true when the children are young or disabled or otherwise experience difficulty explaining their symptoms. As children grow older or become more verbal, they become more capable of active involvement in medical visits. Stivers (2001) examined how physicians, parents, and children negotiate the selection of the next speaker in pediatric encounters. Although doctors most frequently selected children as problem presenters, parents were the most likely actually to present the child's problem. At the same time, parents acknowledged their child's right to answer direct questions. Thus, if the physician directly asked the child a question, the parent typically allowed the child to answer.

However, research has shown that even though communication with children improves adherence and satisfaction (Holzheimer, Mohay, & Masters, 1998; Stebbing, Wong, Kaushal, & Jaffe, 2007), the child typically contributes only minimally to conversations with physicians. Tates and Meeuwesen (2000) videotaped more than 100 medical interviews over a period of almost 20 years. Overall, physicians spoke 51% of the time, parents 39%, and children 9%. In addition, the researchers found that physicians seldom addressed children directly (13% of turns) and parents did so even less (5%). Physicians addressed older children (10–12 years) more than younger children (4–6 years), but parents, interestingly, did not.

Both physicians and parents behave in ways that inhibit child participation. Tates, Elbers, Meeuwesen, and Bensing (2002) found that physicians explicitly invited the parent to formulate the problem and discussed diagnostic and treatment information only with the parent. Parents tended to speak for their children, either by ignoring the child's contribution or interrupting physician–child interactions. On the whole, neither physicians nor parents provided much support for child participation; rather, the child was treated as a passive bystander. In particular, during the diagnosis and treatment portions of the discussion, the child's voice was left out. In essence, all three participants construct an understanding of the nature of the conversation. Parents take responsibility, which is hardly ever questioned by children. Physicians ratify this arrangement by focusing primarily on parents.

Less is known about medical communication with children with disabilities. Although there has been considerable discussion of the rights of children with disabilities in health care decisions (see, for example, J. Davis & Watson, 2000), there is little empirical evidence pertaining to their participation in medical decision making. Young, Moffett, Jackson, and McNulty (2006) examined the role of children with cerebral palsy in medical decision making regarding therapy services in England. Children were less involved in decision making than their parents, and their role was primarily limited to how interventions were implemented. Garth, Murphy, and Reddihough (2009) conducted a qualitative study of communication between physicians, parents, and children with cerebral palsy in Australia. The child was not perceived to be an equal in the conversation.

Shilling, Edwards, Rogers, and Morris (2012) conducted a systematic review of the literature on the experiences and participation of children with disabilities in medical decision making pertaining to inpatient hospital stays. They found that children and parents both identified communication between nurses and patients as a key factor in defining a "good nurse." A good nurse was one who made children feel special and brave and who listened to them. In addition, children appreciated nurses who explained medical procedures to them but were upset when they were excluded from information and decision making. Parents valued nurses who attempted to talk directly with their children but often felt that such communication was lacking. Shilling et al. concluded that the care for children with disabilities was not optimal and that communication between children and hospital staff members often constituted a problem. They suggested that training medical staff in communication with younger patients could improve the inpatient experience for both children with disabilities and their families.

Franklin and Sloper (2009) interviewed 76 professionals, 24 parents (or caregivers), and 21 children with learning disabilities regarding the role of children in medical communications. The authors reported that although the participation of children with disabilities in various areas of decision making has increased in recent years, these children were still less likely to be involved in medical decisions than their able-bodied peers. Moreover, significant barriers to participation remain, especially for children with communication impairments.

When children with disabilities are able to participate in medical decisions, they appreciate the opportunity and are able to voice their concerns (Cavet & Sloper, 2004). For example, Noyes (2000) studied hospitalized children who were ventilator dependent, some of whom had communication impairments, and found that they were interested in earlier discharge. However, there is little current evidence that children's preferences directly influence the delivery of services (Franklin & Sloper, 2009).

Impact of Medical Discourse

Does the type of communication between physician, parent, and child make a difference? There is reason to think it does. Two lines of research are relevant. Some ethnographic studies have examined the effect of specific communication processes on the likelihood of physicians prescribing medication. In addition, some research explores the relationship between more global aspects of communication and parent satisfaction.

Consider first the prescription studies. Overt requests for antibiotics are relatively rare (Stivers, 2002a), so the pattern of indirect requests is worth examining. Stivers (2002b) distinguished between two approaches taken by parents in their opening descriptions of their child's medical condition. Sometimes parents use a "symptoms only" presentation in which the parents portray themselves as supplying the relevant patient data to a medical professional who has the expertise to interpret those data (e.g., "She's had a persistent cough for a few days"). Alternatively, parents may present a "candidate diagnosis" in which they state or strongly imply that they would be receptive to a particular diagnosis and treatment (e.g., "We're thinking it might be an ear infection"). Physicians were more likely to perceive parental expectations as favoring antibiotics when they are presented with a candidate diagnosis rather than a symptoms-only presentation. Moreover, physicians' perception of parent preferences influences their prescriptive decisions (Mangione-Smith, McGlynn, Elliott, Krogstad, & Brook, 1999). When physicians thought that the parents wanted an antibiotic for their child, they prescribed them 62% of the time. In contrast, when they believed the parents did not want a prescription, the percentage was 7%. Physician perception of parent expectations influenced physician prescriptions; however, actual parent expectations did not.

Subsequent studies examined the effects of different words that pediatricians use to make treatment recommendations. One delivery format that physicians may use is to make an affirmative recommendation for a particular treatment (e.g., "I'll give her some cough medicine"). Alternatively, they may make a recommendation against particular treatment (e.g., "She doesn't need an antibiotic"). Presentation of a specific affirmative recommendation for treatment was less likely to receive parental resistance for a non–antibiotic treatment recommendation than for a recommendation against a particular treatment (Stivers, 2005). Thus, parents participate in the treatment decisions regarding their children—even if at times covertly—through their acceptance of or resistance to physicians' treatment recommendations.

Sometimes small changes in communication make a difference. Heritage, Robinson, Elliott, Beckett, and Wilkes (2007) contrasted the choice of *some* versus *any* in the questions that physicians posed to patients (e.g., "Is there something else you want to discuss today?" vs. "Is there anything else you want to discuss today?"). When physicians used *some*, a significant reduction was found, relative to a control condition, in patients' unaddressed concerns, defined as those concerns listed on previsit surveys but not addressed during the office visit. When they used *any*, no reduction was found. Similarly, answers to the question "What can I do for you today?" were four times as long as responses to the question "Sore throat and runny nose for two days, huh?" (Heritage & Robinson, 2006). Thus, when physicians asked more open-ended questions, they received fuller responses from patients, and fewer concerns were unaddressed.

Looking at communication at a more global level, Nolan et al. (2007) examined the role of communication in accessing services and medical equipment for children with developmental disabilities. As noted earlier, most families had no problem in securing acute care and therapy services;

however, almost half of the families reported difficulty in obtaining medical equipment. Moreover, the communication with medical professionals made a difference. Families who reported better communication with their child's primary care physicians had less difficulty in obtaining medical equipment.

Galil et al. (2006) assessed the level of parental satisfaction with child development services as a function of parent–physician communication. Parents of children with a variety of developmental disabilities completed a 15-item questionnaire that measured parental satisfaction regarding communication with the center's physicians. Results of factor analysis revealed that caring (e.g., providing emotional support), interest (e.g., interest in the child's home life), and collaboration (e.g., the physician's willingness to hear the family's opinion rather than dictating the treatment) were positively and significantly correlated with parental satisfaction. The correlation between collaboration and parent satisfaction was the strongest ($r = .64$). A multiple regression analysis found that collaboration was the only significant predictor of parent satisfaction. These results are consistent with the notion that parents are interested in partnering with their child's physicians to secure medical services for their children. A second study comparing satisfaction in two groups of Israeli parents (Jews and Bedouins) also found that parent satisfaction was closely related to the degree of collaboration between parents and health care providers (Bachner, Carmel, Lubetzky, Heiman, & Galil, 2006).

Parish, Magaña, Rose, Timberlake, and Swaine (2012) examined the utilization and quality of health care in Latino children with ASD and other developmental disabilities. Compared with White children, Latino children had worse health care access, utilization, and quality. Moreover, Parish et al. found that the quality of provider interaction mediated the relationship between ethnicity and health care utilization. In particular, three of four quality indicators—provider does not spend enough time with the child, provider is not culturally sensitive, and provider does not make parent feel like a partner—were significant mediators. Thus, certain aspects of the quality of the communication between providers and parents had an impact on parents' utilization of health care services.

At least one targeted intervention has shown promising results. Weiss, Goldlust, and Vaucher (2010) assessed the satisfaction of parents with infants in the newborn intensive care unit (NICU) before and after an intervention aimed at improving communication between parents and medical providers. The intervention educated providers about family communication, distributed contact cards to families, and showed a poster of providers in the NICU. The intervention improved parent satisfaction with provider communication.

Although the Weiss et al. (2010) study is promising, more comprehensive efforts at assessing parent satisfaction with their NICU experience are needed. In light of the earlier studies suggesting a link between parents' immediate experience in the NICU and posttraumatic stress disorder, longer-term studies of parent–provider communication would be particularly appropriate.

Some conclusions are in order. It is clear that the quality of health care that children receive depends in part on the success of the parent in securing appropriate services and equipment from medical providers. This success, in turn, is related to parents' ability to communicate effectively with medical professionals. As we have seen, the nature of this communication can be subtle. Although physicians traditionally operate from a position of authority, many are willing to listen carefully to parents when making treatment decisions. For their part, parents are sometimes distressed by the manner in which physicians refer to their children with disabilities or dismiss parental concerns. However, parents also understand that physicians can make a difference in their child's health. On the whole, physicians and parents are partners who play different roles in negotiating appropriate health care for children with developmental disabilities.

One obvious limitation of this line of research is that a relatively small percentage of the research has been conducted on families with disabilities. Although studies of antibiotic prescription behavior are clearly relevant for the population of children with special health care needs, additional studies of communication between parents of children with disabilities and their children's physicians covering a broader range of topics would be beneficial.

In Chapter 6, I turn to another microsystem: the educational system.

6

SPECIAL EDUCATION, INCLUSION, AND ADVOCACY

Kids who are in the special ed program are off in one wing of the school and kids who are in a so-called regular ed program are off in another wing. What message do you get? (Soodak & Erwin, 1995, p. 266)

The transition of children with disabilities to formal schooling introduces new challenges and responsibilities for their parents. Parents are interested in securing the most appropriate educational environment for their children, which is often although not always an inclusive approach. Not infrequently, educators respond that the cost of providing services for all children with disabilities can be burdensome for school districts with limited or declining budgets. Moreover, educators express reasonable concerns that if the frequencies of conditions such as autism spectrum disorder (ASD) continue to increase, the number of students requiring services will rise even further in the coming years (Mandlawitz, 2002). As a consequence, securing educational services for children with disabilities often requires their parents to take on a new role as educational advocates.

This chapter focuses on parents' perspective on their child's education: what parents want and expect, what they do to try to make that happen, and

http://dx.doi.org/10.1037/14192-006
Families of Children With Developmental Disabilities: Understanding Stress and Opportunities for Growth,
by D. W. Carroll

ultimately how satisfied they are with their child's educational experience. I begin by looking briefly at the laws pertaining to the education of children with disabilities and discuss the range of ways in which these laws may be implemented. I then consider the attitudes of educational professionals and parents and discuss common ground and points of difference. I next discuss how parents become advocates for their children with disabilities and the sources of conflict and collaboration between parents and educational professionals. Finally, I review studies that assess parents' satisfaction with their child's education.

LEGAL PROTECTIONS FOR CHILDREN WITH DISABILITIES

The historical background on the legislative action that provides legal protections for children with disabilities is covered by many sources (Harris, 2010; Martin, Martin, & Terman, 1996; Turnbull, H. R. III, Wilcox, & Stowe, 2002; Yell, Rogers, & Rogers, 1998). I will not review them fully here; however, some brief historical observations are in order.

Through much of the 20th century, children with disabilities were routinely marginalized or even excluded from the public schools. In 1919, a Wisconsin Supreme Court ruling held that a child with a condition that caused facial distortions and drooling could be excluded from school on the grounds that his condition required too much teacher time and nauseated both the teacher and the students (Yell et al., 1998). Beginning in the late 1960s and early 1970s, parents and advocates for individuals with disabilities began to use the court system to force states to provide equal opportunities for these students. These efforts led to the passage of federal legislation that ensured the educational rights of children with disabilities.

The first major effort to protect individuals with disabilities came in 1973, when Congress passed Section 504 of the Rehabilitation Act. Mirroring other civil rights laws, Section 504 prohibited discrimination on the basis of handicapping conditions. Two years later, President Gerald Ford signed Public Law 94-142, the Education for All Handicapped Children Act, which required states to implement policies that would ensure a free and appropriate public education for all children with disabilities to receive federal funds. The law also mandated that schools provide individualized educational plans for students with disabilities and outlined administrative procedures that enabled parents to dispute decisions that were made concerning their child's education.

The title of the act was changed in 1990, when President George H. W. Bush signed the Americans With Disabilities Act into law. The education portion of the act, now called the Individuals with Disabilities Education

Act, identified students with autism and traumatic brain injury as a separate and distinct class entitled to the law's benefits (Yell et al., 1998). In addition, the act mandated transition planning for all students 16 years old or older. Finally, the language of the legislation changed to emphasize the person rather than the disability (*individual with a disability* rather than *handicapped student*).

These legislative efforts have been successful in that overt discrimination is no longer legal, and the number of children with disabilities served in the public school system has increased substantially since the 1970s (Lewit & Baker, 1996). The legislation has laid out procedural protections regarding eligibility for special education services, parental rights, and individualized educational programs. Moreover, the legislation has required that children with disabilities be educated in the least restrictive environment, meaning that they should have the opportunity to be educated with their nondisabled peers to the greatest extent appropriate.

Despite these successes, the legislation leaves some important questions unanswered. Paramount among them is the question of who determines the educational placement of a child (i.e., regular classroom or special education classroom). The regulations provide little guidance other than the stipulation that a student's parents must be involved in the process (Yell & Katsiyannis, 2004). The failure of legislation to speak to this issue has had several consequences. For one, implementation of these legislative acts varies significantly from state to state (MacFarlane & Kanaya, 2009). For another, the ambiguity of the legislation requires parents and educational professionals to work together to determine the most appropriate educational placement for children with disabilities.

ATTITUDES OF PARENTS AND EDUCATIONAL PROFESSIONALS

Some authors have suggested that parents and teachers are necessarily at odds with one another and that parents can be "difficult" when they have "unrealistic" expectations for their children. This is an overly simplistic view. Parents and teachers can be effective collaborators, each playing different yet complementary roles in the education of students with disabilities. However, the roles are not always congruent. Parents sometimes have attitudes that teachers and principals may find challenging, and vice versa.

Parental Views on Inclusive Education

Let us begin with some definitions. *Inclusion* is an arrangement in which children with special needs spend between half and all of their school day in the general education classroom. *Mainstreaming* is one in which children receive consistent part-time placement with general education students. *Special education* refers to an educational placement in which students with disabilities receive their education in a different classroom than, and have little contact with, general education students. In other words, the three arrangements exist on a continuum defined by the amount of time children with special educational needs spend with general education students.

The distinction between inclusion and mainstreaming has evolved over the years. Mainstreaming typically means that the child, although spending much of the school day in the regular education classroom, has a special education classroom as the home classroom. In many situations, children who are mainstreamed are often placed in the general education classroom without appropriate support services needed for educational success. Mainstreaming may be reserved for less academically rigorous courses, such as physical education, or for children with less significant disabilities who are regarded as able to "keep up" with regular education students. Inclusion, in contrast, is a broader concept that is based on the child's right to be educated with one's peers and the school's duty to accept the child. Inclusion typically is understood as requiring the provision of curricular adaptations and support in the form of teaching assistants, trained peer tutors, or interpreters.

Parents of children with disabilities generally endorse inclusion. For example, Elkins, van Kraayenoord, and Jobling (2003) found that 96% of parents of children with disabilities agreed or strongly agreed that children should be given every opportunity to function in the regular classroom. Most also agreed that including a child with special needs in regular education classes promotes the child's independence and that the presence of children with special needs fosters acceptance of difference by other students. These parents favored inclusion even while they recognized that it would require significant changes in the regular classroom as well as additional training for teachers.

However, parental support for inclusion is not unconditional. Kasari, Freeman, Bauminger, and Alkin (1999) found that parents of children with Down syndrome were likely to endorse inclusion as the ideal placement for their child, whereas parents of children with autism were more likely to endorse mainstreaming. Parents of younger children and parents whose children were already placed in general education programs were more positive toward inclusion than were parents of older children or those in special education classrooms. Similarly, Palmer, Fuller, Arora, and Nelson (2001) found that parents differed on whether inclusion was appropriate for all children or their own children. Parents who were supportive of inclusion believed that the child would learn more in a general education classroom, whereas parents opposed to inclusion indicated that the severity of their children's disabilities precluded any benefit from such programs. Parents opposed to inclusion were also concerned that both teachers and students in general education classes would not be welcoming to their children. Thus, although parents generally endorse inclusion, they also recognize that it may not be the most appropriate placement for all children with disabilities.

Attitudes of Educational Professionals

Many teachers and other educational professionals appreciate the value of inclusion but have reservations regarding how to implement legislative mandates. Others are opposed to inclusion. Lawson, Parker, and Sikes (2006) examined narratives of teachers and teaching assistants about inclusion. One of the themes that emerged from the narratives was a sense of ambivalence derived from the practical difficulty of implementing inclusion. One assistant said the following:

> I mean, autistic spectrum disorders, dyslexia, dyscalculia, you can go on forever, but in the time restrictions of this school, I mean, when you think that you're a teaching assistant and you have 20 other children in that class. In the class that I work in there are six, approximately six, children with special needs. When one child needs that amount of input, you have to question whether inclusion is working for that particular child. Sorry. (Lawson et al., 2006, p. 60)

Other teaching assistants were also ambivalent, believing that it was important for children with special needs to be included in the school (as opposed to an institution), but not necessarily in the general education classroom.

Similarly, Agran, Alper, and Wehmeyer (2002) found that most teachers they surveyed did not believe that regular classroom placement was appropriate for a child with severe disabilities. They also did not think that such children should be held to the same academic standards as their nondisabled peers: 48% of teachers disagreed and 40% strongly disagreed that students with moderate to severe disabilities should be held accountable to the same performance standards as typically developing children. The teachers supported access to the general curriculum for students with mild disabilities, but they preferred alternative assessment procedures for students with severe disabilities. Although the teachers surveyed were aware of the federal mandate to ensure access for all students, they did not believe that it had much relevance for students with severe disabilities.

Gilmore, Campbell, and Cuskelly (2003) examined knowledge about Down syndrome and attitudes toward inclusion in a large sample of experienced teachers ($n = 538$) and community members ($n = 2,053$). Both groups significantly underestimated the average life expectancy of a person with Down syndrome and revealed a positive stereotype that a person with Down syndrome was particularly affectionate and happy. Moreover, despite their recognition of the academic and social benefits of inclusion, only about 20% of teachers believed that the regular education classroom was the best setting for children with Down syndrome; teachers were more favorable to the view that children with Down syndrome should be taught in classes with students of a similar developmental level. The views of community members were similar to those of the teachers.

Several studies have examined variables that influence teacher acceptance of inclusion (Podell & Soodak, 1993; Soodak & Podell, 1994; Soodak, Podell, & Lehman, 1998). Teachers with higher levels of self-efficacy were significantly more receptive to inclusion than those with lower self-efficacy, who were more likely to (inappropriately) regard socioeconomic status as a factor in educational placement. Soodak and Podell (1994) gave teachers a case study and asked them to indicate what they believed to be the cause of the student's difficulties, how the needs of the student might be met, and which suggestions they believed would be effective. Teachers most often suggested strategies based on factors other than teacher behavior. Teachers who had greater personal efficacy made more teacher-based strategies, whereas teachers with lower personal efficacy sought solutions elsewhere. Teachers tended to attribute the student's problem to home causes, and their causal beliefs were related to the type of strategies they offered.

Given the gap between the views of parents and professionals that sometimes exists, Cole's (2005) study of mothers of children with disabilities who are also teachers is particularly informative. The mother–teachers had a greater concern that there was good faith and effort on the part of educators than with any particular educational approach. They wanted to be welcomed into either a special school or a mainstreamed school. Although these parents recognized the value of inclusion, they also spoke of the need to find the right balance between the philosophy of inclusion and the reality. Cole summed up these reflections:

> For these mother–teachers inclusion is not about quick fixes or certainties but about shared willingness and commitment to try. It is not about grand rhetoric but the small detail of everyday lived experience. The mother–teachers here are willing to take risks in different ways, as teachers and mothers, on behalf of their own and their "other" children, but these have to be taken within a system which cares for and about their children and has something to offer them in return for the risks they take. Emerging from their voices is the plea that we should not dismiss inclusion because it takes time to get it right or because we make mistakes along the way, but that as educational professionals, parents, and community, we persevere with "good faith and effort" to ensure that ultimately the "risk" of inclusion is one which is worth taking. (p. 342)

These mother–teachers provided nuanced views of educational inclusion that recognized the rights of children with disabilities but also the practical difficulties of implementing legislative mandates. They acknowledged that the issues associated with the inclusion of students with disabilities could be complex and the need for parents and teachers to develop trust and good faith in one another.

A small number of studies have examined the attitudes of principals. Praisner (2003) surveyed elementary school principals' attitudes toward inclusion and found that most of the principals were uncertain about inclusion but were largely favorable. Principals with more positive experiences with students with disabilities and those with more in-service training possessed more positive attitudes toward inclusion. Principals with more positive attitudes and experiences were more likely to place students in less restrictive, more inclusive settings.

K. Callahan, Henson, and Cowan (2008) compared the attitudes of parents, teachers, and administrators regarding the inclusion of children with autism. Similarities on most of the items were found, including attitudes toward the value of an individualized educational plan. However, a few differences in perceptions were found. For example, parents were more likely than educators to believe that there should be observation rooms or windows to allow parents and other professionals to observe the classroom unobtrusively. They were also more likely to believe that parents should have meaningful, active involvement in every stage of the educational planning process, that students should be provided with an intensive treatment program for a minimum of 25 hours per week, and that schools should use student-to-teacher ratios equal to three students to every adult to permit students to achieve individualized instructional goals. Parents placed more emphasis on traditional academic content areas, such as math, reading, and writing, than did teachers of children with autism.

CONFLICT AND COLLABORATION BETWEEN PARENTS AND EDUCATIONAL PROFESSIONALS

Parents of children with disabilities are frequently frustrated by what they regard as insufficient commitment by educational professionals to the goal of inclusive education. As a consequence, some parents have become advocates for educational change in their children's schools, and particularly for greater inclusiveness of students with disabilities. Becoming an advocate is a new role that may require parents to negotiate with and support teachers and to monitor the success of educational programs (Stoner & Angell, 2006). The new role, although an opportunity for personal growth, is often frustrating. As parents have stepped up their advocacy efforts, tensions between parents and educational professionals sometimes become more pronounced.

Parental Concerns and Advocacy

Erwin and Soodak (1995) and Soodak and Erwin (1995) investigated the experiences of nine parents of children with disabilities with regard to how their children's educational placement occurred, how they defined inclusion, their experiences in pursuing inclusive education, and how the process affected them. Although the parents desired inclusive education as a fundamental right for their children, they did not believe that the schools' philosophy and practices necessarily supported the goals they held for their children. In response, they employed a variety of strategies to obtain such education for their children, which included pursuing legal channels, seeking media attention, or moving the family to a new town.

In becoming advocates, some of the parents appeared to discover latent personal skills. They had become more assertive than at any other point in their lives. Some parents remarked that they had never challenged anyone in a position of authority before. Although some of the interactions led to tensions (e.g., parents were regarded as too "pushy"), these parents learned how to negotiate effectively with educational professionals on behalf of their children. They learned that it was necessary to be both assertive and pleasant to work effectively with educators. Erwin and Soodak also noted that the parents became more socially connected: They spread awareness of the need for inclusion and worked with other parents with similar interests.

Swanke, Zeman, and Doktor (2009) studied the emergence of activism in mothers of children with ASD who wrote blogs about their experiences. These mothers expressed considerable discontent with educational, health, and social institutions, including dissatisfaction with the condescending manner in which educational professionals sometimes treated parents. The mothers used blogs as a means of organizing parental responses into a more effective collective response.

Ryan and Cole (2009) explored the distinction between advocacy and activism in mothers of children with ASD. Most of the mothers they interviewed adopted an advocacy role by independently pressing for additional services for their children or working with support groups. A smaller group of mothers demonstrated an activist role in seeking to effect change outside of their families. Many of these mothers expressed concerns about inclusiveness that were broader than school practices. One mother of a 5-year-old put it the following way:

I want him to feel part of society. You know, I want him to, I want people to see him doing things and think he has got a right to be there, because at the moment some people are very sort of sheltered, and they don't think that a disabled child has the right to everything that other children have. And we have had a couple of good talks with people in places like McDonalds when they don't think we have the right to park in a disabled parking place or, you know, that is their view, but he has the right, and it is just trying to educate wider society about the effects of autism as well. (Ryan & Cole, 2009, p. 50)

Thus, for some mothers, interactions with school professionals became the catalyst for assuming a role that extends beyond the school to the wider social world.

Sources of Conflict and Collaboration

Stepping back from the interactions between parents and educational professionals, some studies have explored the sources of conflict and collaboration between parties. Lake and Billingsley (2000) analyzed the factors that contributed to parent–school conflict in special education. Using telephone interviews of parents, school officials, and mediators, the authors identified eight categories of factors that escalate parent–school conflict. These categories included discrepant views of a child or a child's needs, knowledge, service delivery, reciprocal power, constraints, valuation, communication, and trust. The core factor, discrepant views of a child or a child's needs, was associated with the initiation or escalation of conflict in 90% of participant interviews. Parents were often distressed when school officials viewed their children from a deficit perspective, emphasizing what their child could not do instead of what the child could do. This study provided a good framework within which to identify the source of conflicts between parents and educational professionals.

Efforts to define the factors that lead to successful cooperation have also been undertaken. Stoner et al. (2005) examined the role of parent perceptions in conferences with educators with an eye toward determining the factors that enhance or reduce trust. When asked whether they trusted educational professionals, the parents they interviewed responded either negatively or conditionally. Although parents understood that financial realities often played a role in educators' positions, they still questioned the educators' genuineness. The parents often pointed to a particular experience that led to a reduction in trust. At the same time, Stoner and colleagues found that certain practices (such as effective communication, listening to and respecting parental views, and following through on promises) tended to enhance trust. Shelden, Angell, Stoner, and Roseland (2010) extended the discussion of trust to the role of principals. Mothers reported that benevolence, open-ness, and competence were key aspects of principals that increased their level of trust.

O'Connor (2008) studied educational partnerships in Northern Ireland and found similar results. O'Connor suggested that an effective partnership is facilitated by a framework of responsive communication, shared expertise, and active engagement:

> I think the most positive bit for me was the school's reaction. They were very keen to learn, as an institution . . . Niall is the first pupil we've had with this [and] we want to get on top of this and learn. The school really clicked in to, "How can we help?" And that was incredibly positive. (p. 261)

Although O'Connor acknowledged that these results might not be wholly representative of all parents, the study suggested one model of collabora-tion that may lead to effective partnerships between parents and educators.

Cultural issues influence the ease of collaboration between parents and educators. Parents from culturally and linguistically diverse (CLD) groups are often less involved in their child's education than parents from majority groups. Parents may decline to be active participants because of cultural and linguistic barriers between parents and educators. Harry (2008) identified a number of barriers to effective collaboration, including a tendency for educa-tors to view CLD families from a deficit perspective, cross-cultural misunder-standings of the meanings of disability, differential values in setting goals for students, and culturally based differences in caregivers' views of their roles. Jung (2011) noted that although special education law requires parents and educators to collaborate, educators tend to have a lack of respect for parent knowledge of their children, instead valuing—or perhaps overvaluing—more objective, professional sources of knowledge. Similarly, Olivos, Gallagher, and Aguilar (2010) suggested that CLD parents are commonly regarded as recipients of, rather than contributors to, educational policy and practice.

Lasky and Karge (2011) provided suggestions for improving the involve-ment of language minority parents. They included hiring a bilingual parent as a paraprofessional coordinator, instituting a program of home visits, and ESL classes for parents. A particularly salient issue as children with disabilities approach adolescence and youth deals with the cultural aspects of transition planning. Transitional issues are taken up in greater detail in Chapter 8.

However, effective partnerships, once established, also need to be maintained. De Geeter, Poppes, and Vlaskamp (2002) examined the views of parents of children with profound multiple disabilities regarding their rela-tionship with professionals at their child's school. A total of 723 responses to a questionnaire sent to 900 parents in the Netherlands were received. For one group of parents, a method that recognized the parents' expertise assigned them a formal role in developing the child's individual educational program. A second group served as a control group. The results demonstrated that parents as a whole regarded cooperation in a favorable light. However, in a post-test after 1 year, there was no significant difference in levels of parent-reported cooperation between the two groups.

PARENTAL SATISFACTION WITH THEIR CHILD'S EDUCATION

As parents reflect on their efforts and the changes they have seen, how satisfied are they? As we might expect from the above studies, parents' levels of satisfaction vary significantly with a host of factors. Three of these factors are the school climate, the nature of the child's disability, and the age of the child.

Leiter and Krauss (2004) examined parental satisfaction as a function of parental requests for additional services, and the responses to those requests. Analyses of national data indicated that only a small percentage of parents request additional educational services for their children with disabilities. Leiter and Krauss found that among those who made requests, the vast majority encountered significant problems in obtaining additional services. The problems included schools that would not provide additional services as well as those that provided services that the parents considered inadequate. Not surprisingly, those who met resistance were much more likely to be dissatisfied with their children's educators. Leiter and Krauss concluded that it is not the act of requesting services but rather failure to achieve the desired result that predicts parental satisfaction.

On the other hand, parent satisfaction is facilitated by a positive school climate as assessed by parent perception. Laws and Milward (2001) investigated parents' satisfaction with the schooling of their children with Down syndrome. A total of 131 parents of children with Down syndrome ages 4 to 19 years responded to a postal questionnaire. Parental satisfaction was positively correlated with school climate as well as with the parents' perceived involvement in their child's education. MacMullin, Viecili, Cappadocia, and Weiss (2010) explored relationships between parent empowerment, parent mental health, and perceptions of children's educational experiences in parents of children with ASD. Parent empowerment was positively correlated with school communication and the child's relationship with the teacher; parental mental health problems were negatively correlated with both variables.

With regard to the nature of the disability, there are some indications that parents of children with ASD are less satisfied with their child's educational experience than are parents of children with other disabilities. Bitterman, Daley, Misra, Carlson, and Markowitz (2008) found that although children with ASD received more services than children with other disabilities, the parents of children with ASD were less satisfied with the services received. Relative to the comparison group, more parents of children with ASD believed that their child needed more of the services already received or other services not currently received. Similarly, Montes, Halterman, and Magyar (2009) found that parents of children with ASD reported more difficulty in accessing school services and more dissatisfaction with the services than parents of children with other special health care needs.

The age of the child is another variable that influences parental satisfaction with education. There are indications that parental satisfaction is greater when children are younger than when they are older. Spann, Kohler, and Soenksen (2003) studied parents of children with autism. Parental satisfaction was high to moderate in families of younger children (4–5 years), but most parents of older children showed low levels of satisfaction with services. Although the sample size was small, the study provides some evidence that parental satisfaction declines as children move through the educational system. Summers, Hoffman, Marquis, Turnbull, and Poston (2005) reported similar results with a larger sample. A total of 147 parents rated the perceived importance of and satisfaction with 18 aspects of their child and family's relationships with their primary service providers. There were no differences among parents of children from 0 to 3 years, 3 to 5 years, and 6 to 12 years of age in importance ratings. However, parents of older children reported lower satisfaction levels. The difference in parental satisfaction among age groups occurred for all subgroups (e.g., ethnic background, educational background, family income), but it appeared to be particularly strong for single parents.

The decline in parent satisfaction over time likely reflects the struggles many parents experience in obtaining the services they request for their children. In addition, the reduction in satisfaction may reflect emerging concerns regarding the transition of students with disabilities out of the formal education system into the larger society. Many parents of young children experience some respite from 24/7 child care responsibilities when their children enter the formal education system and become eligible for special services. As these children begin to transition out of the public school system, many have ongoing developmental issues coupled with significant uncertainties regarding future education, employment, and independent living. I discuss transitional issues in Chapter 8.

To sum up, in these last two chapters, I have considered how parents interact with and perceive medical and educational professionals. Although there are some similarities in the two cases (e.g., some parents are offended by what they regard as condescending or detached attitudes among professionals and may believe that their views are not taken seriously), there are also some salient differences. Regarding the medical system, parents are most concerned about coordination of care and in determining how to access services and equipment, including learning how to communicate with medical personnel. The issues that parents have with educational professionals appear to run deeper: Many parents distrust teachers and do not believe that teachers have the best interests of their children in mind. The observation that parents are increasingly dissatisfied with their child's education is one indication that relations with the school system are a significant source of stress in the lives of parents of children with disabilities.

In the last three chapters, I have considered three of the microsystems that serve as context for parents of children with disabilities: the family unit, the medical context, and the educational system. In the next chapter, I turn to the macrosystem and examine societal attitudes toward people with disabilities and how these attitudes affect the family.

7

SOCIAL EXCLUSION AND SOCIAL SUPPORT

[She] looked so normal for the longest time. I think that was one of the problems . . . I'd go into a store . . . and someone would say: "For God's sake aren't you spoiling that child. She's awfully big to be carrying"— not knowing that you'd love to put her down, but you can't . . . (Green, 2001, p. 807)

Most children participate in a number of activities in their communities, ranging from church groups to baseball games to trips to the grocery store. Through participation in these activities, children come to feel part of their community and, in particular, connected to their peer group. At the same time, these activities help children eventually appreciate the social and behavioral norms characteristic of their communities.

Children with disabilities have difficulty in conforming to expectations, and their behavior arouses various responses from the general public, including embarrassment, laughter, and anger. As a consequence, some parents may feel their children are not welcome in many situations and choose to reduce their interactions with friends and various social groups. Such social contraction limits the opportunities for parents to receive support as well as to engage in other desired activities besides parenting. This chapter discusses some of the psychological challenges associated with the social exclusion of

http://dx.doi.org/10.1037/14192-007
Families of Children With Developmental Disabilities: Understanding Stress and Opportunities for Growth, by D. W. Carroll

children with disabilities and their families and some of the ways that families respond to these challenges.

In this chapter, I begin by considering the insights of sociologists and social psychologists regarding how certain groups are marginalized in society and how social exclusion influences individuals. Then I examine how children with disabilities and their families respond to societal messages and explore ways of promoting friendship and peer acceptance of children with disabilities. Next, I identify the types of social support that are available to parents of children with disabilities and assess their effectiveness. Finally, I step back and look at the broader picture by examining the global concept of family quality of life.

SOCIOLOGICAL AND SOCIAL PSYCHOLOGICAL PERSPECTIVES

Sociologists and social psychologists have contributed insights on how various groups are marginalized by society as well as the psychological consequences of marginalization. A central concept is stigma.

Stigma

In a seminal book on stigma, Goffman (1963) argued that individuals who have characteristics considered to be undesirable—physical deformity, mental illness, drug addiction, prostitution, and others—are stigmatized or devalued by society. Such individuals are regarded as not quite human, and societies develop terms (e.g., "bastard," "moron") to designate them as such. Moreover, Goffman suggested that individuals who are associated with a stigmatized individual, such as family members, are given what he referred to as a *courtesy stigma*. The problems of the stigmatized person spread out in waves of diminishing intensity. Goffman observed that individuals with courtesy stigmas sometimes have an uneasy relationship with both the stigmatized groups and the people who stigmatize them, since they are not truly members of either group.

These social designations often make interactions between the stigmatized individual and other members of society awkward. Stigmatized persons may feel as if they are being closely watched and need to be careful about the impression they are sending. For example, Goffman wrote of ex–mental patients who had to be vigilant about having sharp interchanges with an employer because of how such a show of emotion might be interpreted. Even when members of society try to act favorably toward a stigmatized person, their actions can be inappropriate; an example would be when conversational partners shout at a blind person.

Psychological Consequences of Social Exclusion

When individuals are stigmatized, they are excluded from many aspects of society. A number of laboratory studies have documented the psychological consequences of social exclusion. Baumeister, Twenge, and Nuss (2002) examined the effects of social exclusion on cognitive processes. Undergraduate students completed a personality inventory and then received false feedback in one of three randomly assigned conditions. In the future-alone condition, they were informed that their test results indicated they were likely to be alone in the future. Another group was told that they were likely to be surrounded with a group of people that cared about them. A third group was told they would be accident prone; this provided a condition with aversive consequences not related to belongingness. The results indicated that the future-alone group showed a large decline in complex cognitive tasks, such as logical reasoning, relative to the other two groups, although no group differences were found in more simple cognitive tasks.

Other studies using this paradigm have found that social exclusion is associated with impairments in self-regulation (Baumeister, DeWall, Ciarocco, & Twenge, 2005) along with increases in both lethargy (Twenge, Catanese, & Baumeister, 2003) and aggressive behavior (Twenge, Baumeister, Tice, & Stucke, 2001). A common theme in these studies is that social exclusion impairs a person's ability to control various impulses. With regard to aggression, Twenge et al. (2001) suggested that people have aggressive impulses that are ordinarily kept in check, but that social exclusion may weaken these restraints, thus enabling aggressive tendencies to prevail. Similarly, in the study on self-regulation, Baumeister et al. (2005) found that individuals in the future-alone condition quit sooner on a frustrating task. In short, self-regulation is an effortful process that is likely to be less successful when individuals do not see its value or do not have the energy to make the effort.

Social exclusion also leads people to seek out different interpersonal connections. The notion here is that when the satisfaction of an important drive is thwarted, individuals seek alternative means of satisfying the drive. Thus, socially excluded individuals may experience a particularly strong drive to form positive social bonds. Maner, DeWall, Baumeister, and Schaller (2007) found that socially excluded individuals expressed a greater desire to meet new friends and work on tasks with other people. In addition, they formed more positive impressions of other people and assigned greater rewards to new interaction partners. Maner et al. suggested that individuals who experience social exclusion respond to such painful interactions both by withdrawing from specific individuals who have provoked unpleasant encounters and by seeking out new social partners.

SOCIAL EXCLUSION OF FAMILIES WITH DISABILITIES

In this section, I explore the implications of the concept of social exclusion of individuals with disabilities and their families. I begin by examining how society responds to individuals with disabilities, first in terms of the spaces allocated for disabled individuals and then in terms of the attitudes toward the disabled. Next, I consider how families respond to these messages. Finally, I consider how social exclusion influences children, review intervention programs designed to facilitate their social inclusion.

Geography of Disability

Some interesting recent research has explored the *geography of disability*—the ways in which society defines appropriate or inappropriate places for individuals with disabilities. Milner and Kelly (2009) identified attributes of place that provide potential participants an anticipation of being welcome. Individuals with disabilities gravitated toward places where they felt known, where they experienced reciprocity, where their participation was expected, and where they felt psychologically safe. Kitchin (1998) observed that other messages suggested that individuals with disabilities should be segregated from the rest of society, as in segregated schools for the deaf or designated areas for wheelchair users in theaters. Kitchin suggested that disability is not merely socially but also spatially constructed: Much of society is organized to keep disabled individuals in their place.

The manner in which individuals are excluded from participating fully in society varies somewhat with the disability. Individuals with mobility problems are obviously limited in their ability to live and work in areas that are not accessible to them. Other individuals may choose not to go to spaces that are not comfortable for them. For example, in one of the few studies of the geography of disabilities with young adults, Madriaga (2010) examined how college students with Asperger's syndrome identified appropriate and inappropriate spaces within a university setting. These students tended to avoid pubs and student unions because they found the rush of crowds and the level of noise to be deeply uncomfortable. However, avoidance of such common student meeting places tended to foster a sense of isolation in these students.

Matters are somewhat different for individuals who are deaf. Many in the deaf community regard societal views as condescending toward individuals with hearing impairment. In particular, they reject the notion that they need to be "fixed" by the larger society (Lane, 1995). Although deaf people have impairments in hearing, they do not necessarily regard themselves as disabled; to the contrary, they regard themselves as part of a valued linguistic

y deaf individuals are more interested in
n being included in the larger community

of disability holds considerable promise for
en and their families navigate their social
of environments that children appreciate—
he like—and how children with disabili-
l.

ith Disabilities

social psychological concepts might be use-
e of disability. As we saw in Chapter 1, the
l to impairment, is defined socially. *Impair-*
a brain injury, that limits a person's ability
to adapt to life. In contrast, a *disability* is defined by how impairments are
regarded in society. Social psychologists emphasize that behavior is often
compared with some normative ideal and that a single personal characteristic
(e.g., race, gender) may lead to a number of inferences about a person. Thus,
the experience of having a disability is inextricably tied to the judgments of
other individuals in society.

Some research has identified correlates of attitudes toward the disabled.
Ouellette-Kuntz, Burge, Brown, and Arsenault (2010) measured attitudes
regarding the social distance that individuals prefer with regard to individuals
with disabilities (e.g., willingness to go to a competent barber or hairdresser
who has an intellectual disability). Older and less educated participants held
attitudes that reflected greater social distance. Participants who had a close
family member with a disability expressed less social distance, as did participants who perceived the disability to be mild. In another study, Akrami,
Ekehammar, and Bergh (2011) examined the correlation between personality characteristics and attitudes toward people with disabilities. They found
that prejudiced attitudes toward people with disabilities were negatively
correlated with openness and agreeableness.

Not all views toward people with disabilities are negative. Some individuals hold positive views that emphasize the efforts made by individuals
to cope successfully with disabling conditions. But Dunn (2000) argued that
these views also miss the mark because of more focus on disabilities than
abilities. There is insufficient recognition that the disability is but one aspect
of a person's life.

Vilchinsky, Findler, and Werner (2010) assessed attitudes in a novel
way: by presenting individuals with scenarios about encounters with individuals with and without disabilities. Reading a scenario about encountering

a person with a disability led to more negative emotions, followed by a compensatory positive cognitive response. The initial negative response appeared to be largely automatic, as it was not influenced by a person's attachment orientation (degree of avoidance or anxiety regarding close relationships). However, the subsequent positive response was moderated by attachment orientation and was stronger among individuals with more secure attachments. The study suggests a dynamic process of self-regulation involving an initial spontaneous negative emotional response accompanied by a compensatory positive response.

In sum, the attitudes of society toward individuals with disabilities and their families consist of multiple components. Individuals often prefer some social distance from those with disabilities, although the extent of this tendency is contingent on personal variables. In the absence of contact, some stereotyped notions of persons with disabilities may develop and endure. Individuals' initial and somewhat automatic response toward individuals with disabilities tends to be negative, but they try to compensate with subsequent positive responses.

Social Exclusion of Children With Disabilities

Studies of peer friendships in the elementary school years typically employ *sociometric analyses*. Children are first asked to nominate peers whom they like or dislike. On the basis of these nominations, researchers identify children as accepted (high number of likes, few dislikes), rejected (few likes, many dislikes), neglected (few likes or dislikes), or controversial (mixture of likes and dislikes). There is little doubt that friendship and acceptance predict significant developmental milestones. Children who have difficulty forming friends are at risk for failed grades, dropping out of school, and the commission of delinquent offenses (Ollendick, Weist, Borden, & Greene, 1992).

On some occasions, children with disabilities are actively rejected by their peers. Although data are sparse, some authors have concluded that children with disabilities are more likely to be at risk for bullying. Sweeting and West (2001) found that children with a sight, hearing, or speech problem were more likely to be teased or bullied; other investigators have found similar results for children with autism and attention-deficit/hyperactivity disorder (Montes & Halterman, 2007) or Asperger's syndrome (Sofronoff, Dark, & Stone, 2011). Carter and Spencer (2006) reviewed 11 studies published between 1989 and 2003 and found that students with both visible and nonvisible disabilities were more likely to be bullied than able-bodied peers. Reported forms of bullying included name-calling, teasing, physical attacks, verbal aggression, and taking of possessions.

Children with disabilities tend to be neglected and have lower socio-metric standing than their able-bodied peers (Cunningham, Thomas, & Warschausky, 2007). Cook and Semmel (1999) found that peer acceptance was lower for children with severe disabilities than for those with moderate disabilities when their classrooms were heterogeneous (i.e., more students with disabilities, more ethnic diversity). However, some research has found that even children with moderate learning disabilities are rejected more than accepted (e.g., Frederickson & Furnham, 1998).

Odom et al. (2006) examined factors associated with the social acceptance and rejection of preschool children with disabilities. The analysis revealed three clusters associated with social acceptance (awareness–interest, communication–play, friendship–social skills) and two clusters related to social rejection (social withdrawal, conflict–aggression). Socially accepted children tended to have disabilities that were less likely to affect social problem solving and emotion regulation. Odom et al. found that children with speech and language impairments and physical impairments were accepted more often than rejected, whereas children with developmental delays and (especially) autism were more likely to be rejected. These results are congruent with studies of typically developing children that indicate that physical attractiveness, communication skills, and social competence are positively correlated with acceptance, whereas aggressiveness is associated with peer rejection (e.g., Newcomb, Bukowski, & Pattee, 1993).

Guralnick (1999) suggested that the difficulties children with intellectual difficulties have in establishing friendships with peers are related to the often-observed behavioral problems they exhibit but extend to issues pertaining to social competence. Furthermore, these issues persist over time (Guralnick, Neville, Hammond, & Connor, 2007). One intriguing finding is that interactions of children with mild developmental delays with their mothers predicted peer relationships (Guralnick, Neville, Connor, & Hammond, 2003). Peer competence of children with developmental delays was negatively correlated with mothers who adopted a controlling disciplinary style. These results suggest an indirect role for families in establishing peer relationships and are consistent with studies of parent–peer relationships in children without disabilities that have found that authoritative parenting (Deković & Janssens, 1992) and parental encouragement of children's emotional regulation (Parke, McDowell, Cladis, & Leidy, 2006) are positively correlated with children's sociometric status.

Just as parents influence their children's social competence, they may also play a role in facilitating their children's acceptance and friendships. A. P. Turnbull, Pereira, and Blue-Banning (1999) discussed parents' facilitation of their children's friendships. The study showed that mothers actively encouraged friendships by exposing children to a wide array of potential friends, encouraging others to accept the child with disabilities, and making accommodations (e.g., advocating for partial participation in community activities).

Promoting Peer Acceptance and Friendships

In addition to exploring the psychological consequences of social exclusion, studies in social psychology suggest ways of fostering positive attitudes toward individuals with disabilities. McManus, Feyes, and Saucier (2011) examined the extent to which contact with and knowledge of individuals with intellectual disabilities predicted attitudes toward those individuals. College students rated their quality and quantity of contact with individuals with intellectual disabilities and their knowledge about intellectual disabilities, and they completed a measure of attitudes toward individuals with disabilities. The results indicated that knowledge about disabilities and quantity of contact did not influence attitudes. However, greater quality of contact was associated with more positive attitudes. The results are consistent with the notion that attitudes are primarily emotional and that positive emotional experiences may lessen intergroup anxiety, hostility, and avoidance.

These results imply that intervention programs that focus on quality of contact are likely to be effective. Current evidence provides some support for this hypothesis. Guralnick, Connor, Neville, and Hammond (2006) reported on a comprehensive intervention program that included both family and school components. Outcome measures emphasized the generalization of peer interactions in unfamiliar playgroups. Results suggested that the effect of the intervention was modest and preventive. Recreational programs also have the potential to promote social inclusion. For example, Siperstein, Glick, and Parker (2009) examined the social acceptance of children with mild intellectual disabilities in a summer recreational program. Peers accepted children with and without disabilities equally. Moreover, 95% of the children without disabilities said they would like to "hang out" with a child with an intellectual disability.

Favazza, Phillipsen, and Kumar (2000) examined the efficacy of a well-designed intervention program to promote peer acceptance of kindergarten children with various disabilities. The 6-week program included three components: a guided discussion group in which children received information about children with disabilities in a regular story period, a structured play component, and a home component in which an adult family member used the same guided discussion technique used at school. Children exposed to individual components showed short-term gains, whereas children exposed to the whole intervention program had both short-term and long-term gains that persisted for 5 months.

SOCIAL EXCLUSION OF FAMILIES

Having a child with a developmental disability often isolates the entire family. DeGrace (2004) interviewed parents of children with severe autism. Several of these children had stringent patterns of routine that made family outings difficult or impossible. Parents indicated that if they drove to church and the child refused to get out of the car, they had little choice other than to simply go home. On other occasions, if the family wanted to go to the mall and the child simply dropped to the floor, the family did not go out. Similarly, Fox, Vaughn, Wyatte, and Dunlap (2002) reported that parents often were afraid to bring their children with disabilities to other people's houses because they were not certain how their children would react.

Social isolation is exacerbated by the responses of other people. A. P. Turnbull and Ruef (1997) report that many parents feel that an ordinary social outing, such as a trip to the grocery store, is uncomfortable because parents do not feel welcome:

> One time I took George to the supermarket, and he kind of jumped up and down and rocked and hummed. He was laughing a lot, and a woman gave me a look. She wouldn't dare say anything, but she gave me a look almost to say, "Why would you bring a boy like that in here?" She didn't have to say anything. Her look told it all. (p. 217[1])

Parents understandably grow reluctant to venture into their communities when they often encounter similar reactions.

Some parents have commented directly on the stigma associated with having a child with a disability. J. Gill and Liamputtong (2011) conducted a qualitative study of mothers of children with Asperger's syndrome. The mothers drew a distinction between children with Asperger's syndrome and other, more publicly visible conditions, noting that people are often more understanding and willing to help a child who is deaf, blind, or wheelchair bound. In contrast, children with Asperger's syndrome who have behavioral issues evoke less sympathetic responses. In light of their children's "normal" appearance but unusual behavior, mothers felt stigmatized in the way that others viewed both them and their children. One mother put it this way:

> To go out somewhere is a nightmare. He can't organize his clothes and doesn't care about grooming standards, so I guess in public it reflects back on me as his mother. . . . Grooming, or lack of, is an embarrassment. (Gill, J., & Liamputtong, 2011, p. 715)

---

[1]From "Family Perspectives on Inclusive Lifestyle Issues for People With Problem Behavior," by A. P. Tumbull and M. Ruef, 1997, *Exceptional Children*, 63, p. 217. Copyright 1997 by Council for Exceptional Children. Reprinted with permission.

Another mother said the following:

> I am a single mother, and all of his bad behavior is always attributed back to his home life, and that was exacerbated by the fact that I am a single mother. . . . I was insulted that I was the stereotypical single mother that didn't put any values into my children, that didn't teach them anything. (Gill, J., & Liamputtong, 2011, p., 715)

The authors concluded that mothers of children with Asperger's syndrome receive a courtesy stigma: They are stigmatized by their association with a child with a disability.

Just as the wider social world has difficulty understanding or accepting the experience of families of children with disabilities, parents of children with disabilities sometimes have difficulty appreciating the ordinary life challenges of parents of typically developing children. Green (2001) interviewed mothers of children receiving therapy, one of whom reported the following exchange:

> I think that in some ways it makes it really hard to relate to a lot of people . . . I remember one time. It was one of those weeks when . . . everything was happening and I was completely stressed about everything and we were wondering constantly . . . whether we were making the right choices. I was talking to a friend and she was real stressed about what dress she was going to put on her child to take a picture that day . . . I just thought: "Just put on the dress you have." What was the big deal? It's so hard sometimes to relate and for other people to relate back to you because they just can't comprehend . . . what you're going through (p. 808)

The net result of these transactions is that families of children with disabilities are frequently isolated from the larger community. As a consequence, they often turn to families with similar circumstances for social support.

SOCIAL SUPPORT FOR PARENTS

Thus, in the social arena, families are challenged by the attitudes of others and the difficulties associated with integrating their children into peer networks. Even when parents are successful in facilitating the peer acceptance of their children with disabilities, these successes come with significant effort on the part of the parents who are already balancing multiple demands. It is beneficial and perhaps necessary for parents to receive social support from family members, friends, and other parents of children with disabilities. Informal nonprofessional support that a family member or friend can provide may include information, advice, or more tangible forms of aid such as childcare. Other parents of children with disabilities may be able to share stories that reduce parents' sense of isolation.

Armstrong, Birnie-Lefcovitch, and Ungar (2005) distinguished between two models of how social support may affect the well-being of individuals and families. The main effect model proposes that social support facilitates well-being by integrating an individual into a larger social network. The buffering model suggests that social support protects persons from the potentially adverse effects of stressful events. Armstrong et al. (2005) proposed that the main effect model directly promotes parental well-being, whereas the buffering model both promotes parental well-being and improves the quality of parenting, which, in turn, provide more favorable outcomes for children.

Respite Care

Abelson (1999) documented the need for respite care services in a survey of 574 families of children with developmental disabilities. Parents indicated a need for respite care services in areas including preparing food, grooming, giving medication, bathing, and lifting. Problems of availability of respite services were reported regardless of demography, income level, or extent of disability. MacDonald and Callery (2004) found that families had different types of respite care needs, including short breaks (3–4 hours) provided by the extended family, short breaks provided by an external agency, and overnight breaks. Interviews with parents, nurses, and social workers found some differences in the perception of appropriate respite care services. For example, parents and nurses valued overnight respite outside of the home, whereas social workers preferred forms of respite that did not separate children from their families.

R. I. Freedman, Griffiths, Krauss, and Seltzer (1999) examined patterns of respite use by aging mothers of adults with intellectual disabilities. Despite an increase in the use of respite care over time, more than half of the 275 families studied never used respite care over a period of 4.5 years. Use of respite care was predicted by functional abilities, health of the adult with intellectual disabilities, and greater maternal caregiving burden.

Strunk (2010) systematically reviewed the literature on respite care for families of children with special needs. The review of 15 quantitative and qualitative studies indicated that respite care was associated with significant reductions in parental stress and opportunities for family time with siblings without disabilities. Strunk also observed that respite care might also be considered a proactive intervention for child abuse for those children suffering from challenging behaviors. The need for respite care transcended many differences between families, including degree of disability, family income, and urban versus rural living. In addition, the demand for respite care was greater during the summer months, when school is not in session.

Parent Support Programs

For parents of children with developmental disabilities, social support from other parents who have dealt with similar issues can play a unique and important role. Although family and friends may provide invaluable emotional support, they typically do not possess the personal experience of parenting a child with special needs. Creating relationships with other parents can alleviate a sense of social isolation for parents of children with disabilities.

We may distinguish between two types of support programs for parents of children with disabilities. Parent support groups provide an opportunity to parents to share common concerns in a group setting. Alternatively, parent-to-parent programs typically match a trained parent in a one-to-one relationship with a parent newly referred to the program. Although both of these programs provide emotional and informational support to parents of children with special needs, the approach is somewhat different. I look at each in turn.

Mandell and Salzer (2007) surveyed 1,005 caregivers of children with autism to determine who joined parent support groups. Approximately two thirds of the sample had participated in an autism-specific support group. Both demographic characteristics of the family and child behavior characteristics influenced group participation decisions. Participation was more likely in families with an annual income over $40,000, those living in suburban areas, and those with a college degree. Parents of children with self-injurious behaviors, sleep problems, or severe language deficiencies were more likely to belong. Parents of children with autism were more likely to join than parents of children with Asperger's syndrome.

Assessment of parent support groups has been limited. Shu and Lung (2005) examined the efficacy of support groups in improving the mental health and quality of life of mothers of children with autism. A quasi-experimental pre–post control group design was used. Mothers were assigned to control or intervention groups based on willingness. Data were collected at pretest, posttest, and follow-up. Few differences were found on any variables. Solomon, Pistrang, and Barker (2001) examined mutual support groups for parents of children with disabilities. Parents reported a high degree of satisfaction with the groups and appreciated belonging to a community with similar interests and experiences. In addition, the group encouraged parents to develop a greater sense of control or agency in the world. Parents often spoke of challenges in working with professionals and felt that the information and advice provided by other parents gave them "ammunition" in their "battles" with professionals.

Consider now parent-to-parent programs. Santelli, Turnbull, Marquis, and Lerner (1995, 1997) surveyed participation in and satisfaction with parent-to-parent programs. Parents preferred to be matched with parents of children with similar disabilities and roughly the same age. Parents valued both the emotional support of having someone to listen and understand and the educational support of providing information on the child's disability as well as community resources. Parents also appreciated the availability of the veteran parents when they needed them.

Singer et al. (1999) and Ainbinder et al. (1998) presented quantitative and qualitative assessments, respectively, on parent-to-parent programs in five states. Singer et al. (1999) presented the quantitative data. Researchers assigned parents either to a treatment group or to a waiting list comparison group. After 2 months, the groups were compared on measures of coping, attitude, and progress in addressing problems. Statistically significant gains were demonstrated for the treatment group in feeling better able to cope with their child, viewing their family and personal circumstances in a more positive light, and making progress on goals that are important to them. No changes in parents' feeling of empowerment were observed. Singer et al. (1999) suggested that the evidence supported the view that parent-to-parent programs are an effective component of a comprehensive family support system.

Ainbinder et al. (1998) presented the qualitative results. The study indicated that a successful match is contingent upon the creation of a "reliable ally" in the supporting parents, comprising four main components: perceived sameness, situational comparisons, round-the-clock availability, and mutuality of support. Regarding mutuality of support, parents benefited both in sharing some of their success stories in handling difficult situations and in learning effective techniques from others. Ainbinder et al. also noted that parent-to-parent programs did not work when a lack of perceived sameness or logistical barriers prevented parents from connecting emotionally with one another. They concluded that parent-to-parent programs, if reviewed for quality control, may be an important adjunct to traditional professional services.

Results to date suggest that parent-to-parent programs provide a useful complement to the support families receive from family members, friends, and mental health professionals. Data on the efficacy of parent support groups are lagging, but the evidence to date is supportive. It is clear that social support often reduces parental distress in these families, but the research has not fully integrated the studies with the models alluded to earlier. As a consequence, we do not necessarily know why support aids parents when it does, and therefore how to maximize the effectiveness of the support.

Nonetheless, the appeal of parent support programs is consistent with the conclusions of social psychologists, discussed earlier in the chapter, that socially excluded individuals seek out alternative ways of gaining positive social connections. It is likely that this is one of the reasons why parents of children with autism and other developmental disabilities often join support groups or one-on-one programs: When the society as a whole does not sufficiently value children with disabilities or appreciate the sacrifices of their parents, at least other parents can be supportive and share similar experiences.

FAMILY QUALITY OF LIFE

We have now considered the family as a system and its links to the medical system, and the school system, and the larger social community. Although it is useful for expository purposes to separate the different contexts in which families function, there is also a need to pull together these multiple strands into a more holistic picture of family life. In recent years, the concept of *family quality of life* has gained currency in disability studies. In this section, we discuss the concept, how it is measured, and what studies along this line may tell us about quality of life in families of children with disabilities.

The concept of quality of life has been discussed in the disabilities field for 3 decades (Schalock, 2000). Although different approaches exist, quality of life is commonly agreed to be a multidimensional concept that cannot be reduced to a single attribute. Schalock (2000) suggested that quality of life includes eight life dimensions: emotional well-being, interpersonal relationships, material well-being, personal development, physical well-being, self-determination, social inclusion, and rights. Each of these dimensions, in turn, can be subdivided. For example, the dimension of social inclusion may include community integration and participation, community roles, and social supports. Another core principle is that quality of life is regarded as the same for all people (Cummins, 2005). Although variation will be evident between individuals in the extent to which certain dimensions are valued, the central notion is that a core of essential components of the quality of life are equally applicable to individuals with and without disabilities. In particular, the concept applies not just to a family member with a disability but rather to all members of the family.

As agreement on the construct emerged, questions of methodology gained in importance. Schalock (2004) observed that the multidimensional nature of quality of life necessitated a methodologically pluralistic approach that included both subjective and objective measures. Researchers at the Beach Center on Disability at the University of Kansas created the Family Quality of Life Scale. The current version of the scale (Summers, Poston, et al., 2005) consists of 25 questions in five domains: family interaction (e.g., "My family enjoys spending time together"), parenting ("Adults in my family teach the children to make good decisions"), emotional well-being ("My family has friends and others who provide support"), physical/material well-being ("My family gets medical care when needed"), and disability-related support ("My family member with special needs has support to make progress at school or workplace"). Summers et al. (2007) used the scale to assess the effect of early childhood service programs. Families' ratings of service adequacy were a significant predictor of family quality of life. On the whole, families were more satisfied with their physical/material well-being than their emotional well-being.

The development of another instrument, the Family Quality of Life Survey, has resulted from the collaboration of researchers from a number of countries, including Canada, Australia, Israel, and the United States (Isaacs et al., 2007). The survey collects qualitative and quantitative data on nine areas of family life: health, financial well-being, family relationships, support from other people, support from disability-related services, spiritual and cultural beliefs, careers, leisure, and community involvement. Within each of the nine areas, individuals are asked six questions about the following: importance, opportunities, initiative, attainment, stability, and satisfaction. Werner, Edwards, and Baum (2009) employed the survey to examine family quality of life following out-of-home placement of a family member with an intellectual disability. Most families reported positive emotional changes following placement. Many families, physically or emotionally exhausted prior to placement, experienced a sense of relief, happiness, and hopefulness. However, there was also evidence of lingering guilt and worry.

The construct of family quality of life appears to hold much promise in providing a holistic view of the impact of child disabilities on families. Brown, Schalock, and Brown (2009) suggested that the quality of life concept is responsive to broad societal issues, including the emphasis on community-based services and the rise in consumer empowerment with its emphasis on self-determination. Although the assessment of such a broad concept presents significant challenges, the efforts to date suggest that it is possible to measure the impact of a variety of variables not only on children with disabilities but also on the families that care for them.

To summarize, in Chapters 4 through 7, we considered how children with disabilities affect families in terms of their internal functioning as well as in terms of their interactions with the medical and educational communities and with society at large. As individuals with disabilities move into adolescence and early adulthood, new concerns arise, which will be our focus in Chapter 8.

8

DEVELOPMENTAL DISABILITIES THROUGH THE LIFE SPAN

"What will happen when she grows up, will she be left to destiny? And what will happen then? This is what I think about, but still push aside. I can only take one day at a time." (Roll-Pettersson, 2001, p. 7)

As individuals with disabilities approach adolescence and early adulthood, there are often significant life decisions to consider. For some individuals, the exit from high school means an opportunity to further one's education in a community college or university. Others may be interested in joining the workforce. For still others, residential issues are of primary importance, as adolescents or young adults move from the family home into a community residence. Parents of individuals with disabilities are involved in planning for all of these transitions, and the success of their adult children in new roles is often associated with parents' well-being at midlife.

The first section of this chapter deals with issues in education, employment, and independent living that persons with disabilities face as they prepare for adult roles. Next, I consider changes in the transactions between parents and their adult children, as parents face the task of balancing their concern for protecting their children with respect for their children's

http://dx.doi.org/10.1037/14192-008
Families of Children With Developmental Disabilities: Understanding Stress and Opportunities for Growth,
by D. W. Carroll

emerging autonomy. The third section assesses parent well-being at midlife. Finally, I examine change and stability in the relationships between individuals with disabilities and their siblings.

TRANSITIONS TO ADULT ROLES

Compared with youth without disabilities, youth with disabilities are at risk for a number of adverse outcomes (G. A. King, Baldwin, Currie, & Evans, 2005). Their rate of participation in extracurricular activities, although rising in recent years, is below that of the general population. They are less likely to be employed or to participate in postsecondary education and are at increased risk for social difficulties after high school. Furthermore, students with disabilities, especially emotional disturbance, are overrepresented in the juvenile corrections systems (Quinn, Rutherford, Leone, Osher, & Poirier, 2005).

Several studies have reported trends for youth with disabilities using data from the National Longitudinal Transition Study (NLTS) conducted by the U.S. Department of Education. Blackorby and Wagner (1996) reported that strong gains in employment, wages, postsecondary education, and residential independence for youth with disabilities in their first 5 years following high school were shown in the NLTS data. However, the data also indicated that youth with disabilities continued to lag behind their peers in the general population. Longitudinal outcomes also differed widely by gender, ethnicity, and high school completion status.

Postsecondary Education

Studies of educational outcomes of youth with disabilities following high school reveal considerable variability. Some students prosper in programs that emphasize specific occupational skills as well as continuous support. Others are interested in college and less in immediate work preparation. Still others exit high school without a diploma and are unprepared for any additional formal education.

Wagner and Blackorby (1996) provided an overview of how special education students fare in the transition from high school to work or college. Thirty percent of students with disabilities dropped out of high school and 8% dropped out before entering high school. Postsecondary educational participation was low; 37% of high school graduates with disabilities had attended a postsecondary school. Students with hearing or visual impairments were most likely to attend college. As a group, students with disabilities were more likely to be poor, and when employed, earned less than the comparison group. Placement in regular education, as opposed to special education, had both positive and negative effects. Students with sensory or motor disabilities appeared to benefit from placement in a regular education classroom. However, for many students, more time in regular education was associated with a higher likelihood of course failure, which was a strong predictor of dropping out.

Recent data are somewhat more encouraging. Sanford et al. (2011) reviewed NLTS data and found that young adults with disabilities are increasingly focused on postsecondary education. They are taking more rigorous academic courses in high school, including college preparatory courses such as foreign languages and science. Student success appears related to the particular disability and to student educational experience in high school. Zhang, Katsiyannis, and Kortering (2007) examined performance on exit exams by students with disabilities. Overall, students with disabilities performed more poorly than did typically developing students. Students with learning disabilities or other health impairments performed better than students with emotional or behavioral disorders or educable mental disabilities. Students with disabilities who had been in general education programs were more likely to attend a 4-year college than students who had been in special education programs (Williams-Diehm & Benz, 2008).

Employment Issues for Youth With Disabilities

Sanford et al. (2011) reported that people with disabilities have a much higher unemployment rate than the general population, although the students who had been in general education programs were less likely to be unemployed than the students who had been in special education (Williams-Diehm & Benz, 2008). In the absence of employment opportunities, many youth with disabilities spend their time in sheltered workshops. However, the availability of these workshops varies with the nature of the disability. J. L. Taylor and Seltzer (2011b) examined postsecondary educational activities for young adults with autism spectrum disorder (ASD). Analyses indicated low rates of employment in the community, with the majority of young adults (56%) spending time in sheltered workshops or day activity centers. Young adults with ASD without an intellectual disability were three times more likely to have no daytime activities compared with young adults with ASD who also had an intellectual disability. Individuals placed in open employment, as opposed to sheltered employment, reported significantly higher quality of life scores (Kober & Eggleton, 2005).

Educational programs that focus on specific occupational skills have showed promise for some youths with disabilities. Phelps and Hanley-Maxwell (1997) reported two educational practices that are aligned with better outcomes. They include school supervised work experiences and functionally oriented curricula in which occupationally specific skills, employability skills, and academic skills are systematically connected for students. More recently, Flannery, Yovanoff, Benz, and Kato (2008) examined the effect of short-term occupational training on employment rates and financial well-being in youth with disabilities. In particular, they examined a program that was individually designed, primarily a work site–based curriculum, with a focus on the existing labor market. Results indicated that successful completion of the program was associated with higher wages and more work hours during the first year after exit.

Residential Issues

Many young people have disabilities severe enough to preclude independent living. Sanford et al. (2011) reported that only 36% of young adults with disabilities were living independently at the time of their interview. A challenge for their parents is whether and when to place these youths in a community residential facility. Several studies have examined factors that influence parental decisions to place their children in community facilities. R. I. Freedman, Krauss, and Seltzer (1997) examined aging parents' residential plans (or lack thereof) for adult children with intellectual disabilities. Less than 50% of the parents had made plans, and most thought their children would still be living in their home in 2 years. At a 3-year follow-up, 22% of the families with short-term residential plans had achieved a placement compared with 14% among families without a plan who wanted placement.

Essex, Seltzer, and Krauss (1997) investigated reasons for residential planning and placement among 461 families of adults with intellectual disabilities. They found three distinct profiles. A small number of families viewed placement as a means to foster independence in their children; for these families, residential placement was a normative launching process. A larger group of families considered placement as a result of a mix of caregiving stress and declining parental health. A third group considered residential placement as a proactive way of securing their child's future after they were no longer able to serve as the primary caregiver.

For the most part, families are satisfied with their decisions, particularly over time. Blacher and Baker (1994) examined family satisfaction pertaining to out-of-home placement for children with intellectual disabilities. Residential placement generally followed a gradual buildup of child-related stress. Parents reported high levels of satisfaction with the placement decision and positive family adaptation following placement. Family experiences were not related to the child's age, level of disability, behavioral problems, or the size of the placement facility. Part of the reason for parental satisfaction is that even after placement, there is considerable family contact. Seltzer, Krauss, Hong, and Orsmond (2001) found continuity of family involvement following residential transitions of adults with intellectual disabilities. Mothers were highly involved in the relocation process and had frequent contact and continued emotional involvement with their adult child. Over time, mothers had decreased levels of direct caregiving but were increasingly satisfied with their level of contact and less worried about the future.

Some attention has been given to the experiences of young adults with different types of disabilities. Esbensen, Bishop, Seltzer, Greenberg, and Taylor (2010) compared young adults with ASD and young adults with Down syndrome on variables indicative of independence in adult life. Adults with ASD had less residential independence and social contact with friends, had more limited functional abilities, and exhibited more behavioral problems than did adults with Down syndrome. Moreover, adults with ASD had more unmet service needs and received fewer services than did adults with Down syndrome.

Cultural issues have also received attention. An underlying theme in the many discussions of transitions is the value and necessity of young adults with developmental disabilities becoming independent and self-sufficient. However, the interpretation of independence varies among cultural and ethnic groups. Rueda, Monzo, Shapiro, Gomez, and Blacher (2005) discussed transition models in the Latina culture, which places a greater emphasis on interdependence than independence and on the dangers of the outside world. Frankland, Turnbull, Wehmeyer, and Blackmountain (2004) found that although self-determination is important in the Navaho (Diné) culture, it is operationalized more in terms of interdependence and group cohesion than in the Anglo culture. These observations suggest that in discussions of transitions, it is important for educators to consider the kinds of environments to which these young adults are transitioning.

Individuals with disabilities face considerable challenges in achieving independence during the later adolescent and early adulthood years. Parents have the responsibility of assisting youth in making these transitions while respecting their desire for greater independence. How parents and their children manage these tasks is our next concern.

CHANGES IN PARENT–CHILD TRANSACTIONS

Physical, intellectual, and social changes occur during adolescence and early adulthood that help redefine the parent–child relationship. As children with developmental disabilities move into adolescence, new concerns and opportunities arise. Adolescents typically are accorded a greater degree of autonomy than children, and to some extent this may reduce parental burdens. On the other hand, children with disabilities may not be able to participate in some of the activities typically available for able-bodied adolescents (e.g., driving), and this may lead to increased tension in the family. We have the benefit of two programs of research on adolescents and young adults with developmental disabilities—one on individuals with spina bifida, the other on those with ASD—that have examined the nature of parent–child transactions over time.

Spina Bifida

Spina bifida is a congenital disorder caused by incomplete closing of the embryonic neural tube. Some vertebrae overlying the spinal cord are not fully formed and remain unfused and open. Physical complications include leg weakness or paralysis, bladder and bowel control problems, and skin irritations. Typically, children with spina bifida have diminished urinary and bowel control and often require the use of a wheelchair. Although individuals with spina bifida are not regarded as intellectually disabled in the usual sense of the term, they sometimes suffer cognitive impairments in executive functioning. For example, children and adults with spina bifida may experience difficulties in planning and organizing activities and in selective attention (Rose & Holmbeck, 2007). In addition, children with spina bifida tend to be socially immature and are more dependent on adults for guidance than are their able-bodied peers (Holmbeck et al., 2003). They also have fewer positive social contacts with peers, which may place them at risk for depressive symptoms (Essner & Holmbeck, 2010).

Nonetheless, families of children with spina bifida show considerable resilience. Families of children with spina bifida show lower levels of dysfunction than families with a child with cerebral palsy (Holmbeck & Devine, 2010). Moreover, families of preadolescents with spina bifida experience less conflict than families with able-bodied children on certain issues. For example, Coakley, Holmbeck, Friedman, Greenley, and Thill (2002) examined pubertal timing and family conflict during the transition to adolescence in children with spina bifida. Early maturity was associated with higher levels of conflict and decreases in family cohesion in families with able-bodied children, but perceived pubertal timing had less of an effect on families of children with spina bifida. Sexuality-based conflict may be lower or delayed in families of adolescents with spina bifida due to the generally delayed psychosocial maturity in these adolescents.

Although autonomous behavior may develop more slowly for children with spina bifida, they show growth in independence during the preadolescent years. Friedman, Holmbeck, DeLucia, Jandasek, and Zebracki (2009) studied autonomy development across the adolescent transition in individuals with spina bifida. They found increases in independence from ages 9 to 15, although the adolescents with spina bifida lagged behind their able-bodied peers. Holmbeck et al. (2010) found a similar pattern for friendships: Although children with spina bifida increased the number of friendships as they moved into the adolescent years, they still had significantly fewer friends than did the comparison group.

As preadolescents with spina bifida gain autonomy, there are changes in family patterns that sometimes spill out into conflict. Stepansky, Roache, Holmbeck, and Schultz (2010) studied medical adherence in 70 families with young adolescents with spina bifida. Data were collected in family interaction sessions by using questionnaires. Findings suggested that responsibility for medical regimens transfers gradually from parent to child over time. Family conflict was related to a decrease in adherence over time. The evidence indicates, however, that families adapt to the conflicts that may appear during this period. Zukerman, Devine, and Holmbeck (2011) examined the influence of parental intrusiveness on the achievement of emerging adult milestones (e.g., attending college, achieving employment, establishing romantic relationships) in youth with and without spina bifida. Typically developing youth were more likely to achieve milestones compared with youth with spina bifida, but the differences disappeared when the variable of high school completion was controlled. Parental intrusiveness, executive functioning, socioeconomic status, and intrusive motivation all predicted various milestones. Parental intrusiveness particularly influenced the emergence of romantic relationships. Parents who were more intrusive had children who were delayed in developing lasting romantic relationships.

Kelly, Zebracki, Holmbeck, and Gershenson (2008) discussed the clinical implications of this line of research. Although there is significant variability within the spina bifida population, adolescents with spina bifida are more at risk for stress, depression, and developmental delays that can be exacerbated by parental overprotectiveness. Kelly et al. suggested that interventions should target families that are most at risk (e.g., low socioeconomic status, single parent families). Interventions that target social isolation and independence issues appear to be particularly useful. For example, O'Mahar, Holmbeck, Jandasek, and Zukerman (2010) found that a camp-based intervention led to gains in independence in children, adolescents, and adults with spina bifida. Given the cognitive issues involved, neuropsychological screening is recommended. In addition, some efforts at educating spina bifida children about the nature of spina bifida and providing tools for discussing the condition with their peers may help mitigate the stigmatization of individuals with spina bifida (e.g., Greenley, Coakley, Holmbeck, Jandasek, & Wills, 2006). Finally, interventions for parents that address issues of stress, communication, and autonomy development appear to be appropriate.

Autism Spectrum Disorder

Although behavioral problems in individuals with ASD remain an issue for many individuals as they approach adolescence and young adulthood, the problems diminish over time. Shattuck et al. (2007) examined changes in maladaptive behaviors in adolescents and adults with ASD over a period of 4.5 years. Individuals ranged in age from 10 to 52 years, with a mean age of 22 years. Although many individuals' symptoms remained stable, a larger proportion of the sample showed declines in autistic symptoms and maladaptive behavior. Those older than 31 had fewer maladaptive behaviors and experienced more improvement over time, consistent with the observation that autistic symptoms abate with age.

The extent to which behavioral problems diminish with age is related to the transactions between parents and autistic youth. One type of transaction that has been studied is the level of expressed emotion in the family. As discussed in Chapter 4, *expressed emotion* refers to the emotional climate of a family; in particular, high levels of expressed emotion are defined as high levels of criticism, marked emotional overinvolvement, or both (Hastings & Lloyd, 2007). Hooley and Gotlib (2000) suggested that a diathesis–stress model may explain the relationship between high levels of expressed emotion and various clinical outcomes. For example, individuals with a high risk for disorders such as schizophrenia may have an increased genetic sensitivity to stress.

Within the disability literature, there is an ongoing debate about the direction of effects between expressed emotion and the behavior problems associated with individuals with disabilities. Greenberg, Seltzer, Hong, and Orsmond (2006) studied a sample of 149 mothers coresiding with their adolescent or adult child with autism over an 18-month period. They found that high levels of maternal expressed emotion were related to increased levels of maladaptive behavior and more severe symptoms of autism over time. A subsequent study found that maternal levels of criticism predicted child behavior problems, but not vice versa (J. K. Baker, Smith, Greenberg, Seltzer, & Taylor, 2011). There is less debate concerning the effects of maternal warmth and praise, which has been found to reduce both repetitive behavior symptoms (L. E. Smith, Greenberg, Seltzer, & Hong, 2008) and caregiving strain (Orsmond, Seltzer, Greenberg, & Krauss, 2006).

A different aspect of the environment that influences the development of autistic youth is the set of activities available for them after exiting high school. J. L. Taylor and Seltzer (2010) studied 242 youths with ASD who had recently left high school. Data collected over nearly 10 years indicated overall improvement in autistic symptoms and internalized behaviors but slowing rates of improvement after exit from high school, suggesting that the shift from school to adult day activities was disruptive for these young adults. These investigators concluded that adult day activities might not be as intellectually stimulating as educational activities in school. Similarly, J. L. Taylor and Seltzer (2011a) found an improvement in the mother–child relationship while the autistic youths were in high school but a lack of improvement after high school. The findings provide further evidence that the years after high school exit are a time of increased risk for those with ASD, particularly those with intellectual disabilities and whose families had fewer resources.

What can we conclude about the progression from childhood to adolescence and young adulthood in individuals with spina bifida and ASD? Although additional research on youths with these disabilities is warranted, work to date suggests that the behavioral issues are somewhat different in the two cases. Children and youths with spina bifida have issues with autonomy and psychosocial maturity, which may be related to a tendency for their parents to become overprotective. Individuals with ASD have persistent maladaptive behaviors, such as repetitive behaviors, that are exacerbated by negative expressed emotions by their parents. As children with these disabilities grow into young adulthood, parents who make positive adjustments in their behavior toward their children may see some improvement in the behavior of their children.

PARENTING AT MIDLIFE

Work–Life Balance

For parents of children with developmental disabilities, work outside the home provides not only income but also a sense of identity and an opportunity to develop a social network of friends. However, as discussed in Chapter 4, juggling the demands of work and family life can be a significant stressor for parents of children with developmental disabilities (S. L. Parish, 2006). Although family-friendly policies can help, many parents are limited to part-time jobs for poor wages or are forced to leave paid employment altogether to care for their adolescent or adult children. These issues are especially challenging for women, who often carry the largest burden of home and child care.

The long-term impact of part-time employment can be financially significant. Parish, Seltzer, Greenberg, and Floyd (2004) explored the economic well-being and employment of parents whose children did or did not have developmental disabilities. This longitudinal study collected respondent data at 18, 36, and 53 years of age. Although the two groups were similar at 18 years, they diverged significantly on economic indicators by

53 years. Mothers of children with disabilities were less likely to have continued employment and had lower earnings at 36 years. There was also a trend for them to be less likely to have full-time jobs as their children grew older, and thus they were less likely to have the associated health insurance. Overall, parents of children with disabilities have significantly lower savings and income by midlife than parents of typically developing children.

More recently, Parish, Rose, and Swaine (2010) analyzed United States census data to examine the financial status of parents with coresident children and adults with disabilities. The findings indicated significant financial vulnerability, particularly for younger (less than 45 years) and older (65 years and older) parents. Compared with middle-aged parents (45–65 years), younger and older parents had less income and less net worth. The authors noted that the sharp decline in net worth for older parents signals dire consequences for parents struggling to finance their retirements while continuing to care for their adult children with disabilities.

Parental Well-Being at Midlife

A sizable body of research has examined the long-term consequences of parenting a child with a developmental disability for parents' psychological well-being. Using data from the Study of Midlife in the United States, Ha, Hong, Seltzer, and Greenberg (2008) found that, compared with parents of nondisabled children, parents of children with disabilities experienced significantly more negative affect, significantly more somatic symptoms, and marginally poorer psychological well-being, even after controlling for sociodemographic variables. Mothers did not differ from fathers in their well-being, but older parents were significantly less likely to experience negative effects related to parenting a child with disabilities.

Caldwell (2008) compared the physical and mental health of female family caregivers of adults with developmental disabilities at four age periods: 35 to 44, 45 to 54, 55 to 64, and 65+ years. No differences in physical health were observed across age groups. However, the mental health of midlife (45–54 years) and older (older than 65 years) caregivers was poor relative to national norms. Caldwell (2008) suggested that the reduced mental health of caregivers might be attributable to two significant life transitions: when young adults with disabilities transition to adult life and when adult caregivers are no longer able to provide care for family members. In addition, the research found that poorer mental health was associated with families with greater unmet health care needs.

Several studies have examined differences and similarities between mothers of children with developmental disabilities and other caregivers. In an early study, Krauss and Seltzer (1993) compared older mothers of adults with developmental disabilities with several reference groups: older women not in a caregiving role, women who served as caregivers for older adults, and young mothers who had a child with an intellectual disability. The older mothers of developmentally disabled adults performed as well as or better than the reference groups on measures of depression, life satisfaction, parenting stress, and social isolation. The authors suggest that these mothers had made positive adaptations to their situations. Greenberg, Seltzer, and Greenley (1993) investigated 105 mothers of adult children with mental illness and 208 mothers of adult children with intellectual disabilities. Mothers of children with mental illness reported higher levels of frustration and lower levels of gratification. Adult children's behavior problems were the strongest predictor of maternal gratification, but diagnosis also played a role. The size of the mother's social network, the family social climate, and the child's participation in out-of-home programs also influenced the effect of caregiver stress.

Abbeduto et al. (2004) examined the psychological well-being of mothers of adolescents or young adults with fragile X syndrome, Down syndrome, or autism. On most measures, mothers of individuals with autism had the lowest levels of well-being and mothers of persons with Down syndrome the highest, with mothers of individuals with fragile X syndrome intermediate. The researchers found that the level of behavioral symptoms exhibited by the youth was the most consistent predictor of maternal well-being.

Several variables influence the life satisfaction of aging mothers. Pruchno (2003) found that mothers' caregiving satisfaction was greater when there was greater affection from child to mother, even when the caregiving burden was not affected. Parental coping strategies also influence well-being. Seltzer, Greenberg, and Krauss (1995) compared problem-based and emotion-based coping strategies in mothers of adults with either developmental disabilities or mental illness. Mothers of adults with developmental disabilities had a lower risk of depression when using problem-based coping but not emotion-based coping. Mothers of adults with mental illness did not benefit from either strategy. Perhaps a more productive approach would be accommodative coping, which involves flexibly adjusting one's life goals in response to a persistent problem. Seltzer et al. (2004) investigated coping in parents of adults with a developmental disability, children with a severe mental health issue, and children without a chronic illness or disability. Parents who used accommodative coping had fewer depressive and physical symptoms.

Marital Quality

As noted in Chapter 4, studies indicated that the divorce rate was higher in parents of children with disabilities than in parents of typically developing children. However, the differences were relatively small and may be partially attributable to factors within the family before the child was born. Additional insight comes from studying marital quality and divorce rates over a longer time period. Recently, Hartley et al. (2010) examined the prevalence of divorce in parents of children, adolescents, and young adults with ASD. The comparison group consisted of parents of children without disabilities that were closely matched on variables such as age, ethnicity, and education. Hartley et al. (2010) found that parents of children with ASD had a higher rate of divorce (23.5%) than did the comparison group (13.8%). Moreover, for parents of children with ASD the rate of divorce remained high throughout childhood, adolescence, and early adulthood, whereas divorce decreased when children were over 8 years old in the comparison group.

The finding by Hartley et al. (2010) of a divorce rate nearly twice as high as in the comparison group contrasts with earlier studies that found more modest differences. However, several of the earlier studies examined families of children with various disabilities. The heightened prevalence of divorce in families of individuals with ASD is consistent with studies discussed earlier in the chapter that indicate high levels of stress in these families.

A subsequent study by Hartley, Barker, Seltzer, Greenberg, and Floyd (2011) examined marital satisfaction and parenting experiences of parents of adolescents and adults with autism. Hartley et al. (2011) found that marital satisfaction was an important predictor of parenting experiences, especially for fathers. Other differences between parents were found: Fathers' parenting experiences were more closely related to child characteristics than were mothers', and mothers reported feeling closer to their son or daughter than fathers did. The study indicates that close relationships exist between marital satisfaction and parenting experiences and that the relationships differ between mothers and fathers.

THE CHANGING ROLE OF SIBLINGS

The sibling relationship may be the longest of all human relationships. As parents age, the roles and responsibilities of siblings change. Seltzer, Greenberg, Orsmond, and Lounds (2005) provided an overview of life course studies of siblings of individuals with developmental disabilities and discussed some methodological issues in this area of research. Several studies have examined differences in sibling well-being and changes in sibling relationships over time. In the general population, siblings often show decreased satisfaction with their sibling relationships during adolescence, and adolescents are prone to depressive symptoms. The question is whether having a sibling with a developmental disability adds risk for depressive symptoms over and above the general risk at this age period.

Sibling Relationships and Sibling Well-Being

Several studies have compared siblings of individuals with intellectual disabilities and siblings of individuals with mental illness. Some individuals have diagnoses of both intellectual disability and mental illness (see Borthwick-Duffy, 1994; Whitaker & Read, 2006). Thus, it is somewhat artificial to contrast individuals with one or the other disability. Nonetheless, such a distinction can be useful in that developmental disabilities and mental illness may lead to different psychological responses in individuals and, as a consequence, in their siblings.

Seltzer, Greenberg, Krauss, Gordon, and Judge (1997) found that siblings of adults with intellectual disabilities were more likely to perceive that their brother or sister had a pervasive influence on their life decisions. In addition, siblings of adults with intellectual disabilities, when asked to assess the effects of their sibling on their career and romantic choices, evaluated their sibling as mostly positive; in contrast, siblings of adults with mental illness assessed the effects as mostly negative. Also, siblings of adults with intellectual disabilities displayed better mental health when they had a close relationship with their sibling. In contrast, siblings of adults with serious mental illness fared better psychologically when they perceived a less pervasive impact of their sibling. Seltzer and colleagues (1997) concluded that siblings of adults with intellectual disabilities use emotional intimacy with their sibling as a key to their well-being, whereas siblings of adults with mental illness use psychological distance to achieve well-being.

Studies also indicate that siblings of adults with Down syndrome generally fare better than siblings of adults with ASD. Orsmond and Seltzer (2007) found that siblings of adults with ASD had less contact with their brother or sister, reported lower levels of positive affect in their relationship, and felt more pessimistic about their sibling's future than siblings of adults with Down syndrome. For siblings of adults with ASD, a closer sibling relationship was observed when the sibling had lower educational levels, lived closer to the sibling with ASD, used more problem-focused coping strategies, and when the sibling with ASD had a higher level of functional independence.

Orsmond and Seltzer (2009) examined predictors of depressive and anxiety symptoms in siblings of individuals with ASD. They collected data from 57 siblings and their mothers. Sisters reported higher levels of depression and anxiety than brothers. A family history of ASD was correlated with depressive but not anxiety symptoms. Moreover, a high level of maternal depression was associated with both depressive and anxiety symptoms. Orsmond and Seltzer (2009) concluded that their results provided some support for the diathesis–stress model; sibling subthreshold characteristics of autism coupled with high levels of family stress predicted depressive symptoms in siblings. These results converge with those of Ingersoll and Hambrick (2011) and Ingersoll, Meyer, and Becker (2011), discussed in Chapter 4, that subthreshold characteristics of ASD (i.e., broader autism phenotype) in mothers of children with ASD served as a risk factor for depression.

Continuity and Change in Sibling Relationships Over Time

There is both stability and change in sibling relationships over time. As adolescents move into adulthood, they often maintain close connection with their siblings with intellectual disabilities. However, the nature of the relationship shifts as their parents grow older and become less able to care for disabled adults. Siblings thus must think about taking over some of these responsibilities.

Several studies indicate that siblings of adults with intellectual disabilities often maintain high levels of involvement with their brother or sister. Krauss, Seltzer, Gordon, and Friedman (1996) examined current relationship patterns and future role expectations of 140 adult siblings of a brother or sister with an intellectual disability still living in the family home. As adults, siblings maintained contact with and provided emotional support for their siblings and felt knowledgeable about their sibling's needs. Many of the siblings lived within 30 minutes of their brother or sister and visited at least weekly. Of those respondents with firm plans for the future, 36% planned to live with their sibling and 64% planned to live apart. Sisters were more likely than brothers to coreside with their siblings.

Again, it is productive to contrast intellectual disability and mental illness. Greenberg, Seltzer, Orsmond, and Krauss (1999) compared present support and future plans of siblings of adults with intellectual disabilities and those with mental illness. Both groups of siblings provided instrumental support to their siblings, but siblings of adults with intellectual disabilities provided significantly more emotional support. Moreover, almost 60% of the siblings of adults with intellectual disabilities expected to assume primary caregiving responsibility in the future, whereas only one third of the siblings of adults with mental illness held this expectation. The stability of sibling relationships was indicated by the finding that the quality of emotional closeness during adolescence was a significant predictor of the expectation of future caregiving responsibility.

Skotko and Levine (2006) noted that most adult siblings of individuals with Down syndrome assume a position of advocacy at some point. Early in life, siblings often encounter challenges such as what to do when other people make fun of one's brother or sister and may need to correct the disparaging language of a classmate. In adult life, some siblings ultimately select a career that is related to children with developmental disabilities. Marks, Matson, and Barraza (2005) interviewed seven individuals who chose a career in special education in part because of their experiences growing up with a brother or sister with a disability. These siblings felt a strong sense of responsibility for their sisters and brothers. Their choice of career was related to a desire to improve services for individuals with disabilities; as a group, they strongly supported inclusion of students with disabilities into the regular education classroom.

Burke, Taylor, Urbano, and Hodapp (2012) conducted a study to determine predictors of future caregiving by adult siblings. A total of 757 siblings completed a 163-item survey that assessed their expectations regarding future caregiving. Siblings who were female, had a closer relationship with their sibling, and were the lone sibling expected to assume greater caregiving responsibilities in the future. In addition, siblings who had parents who were currently more able to care for their brother or sister with a disability expected to assume higher levels of caregiving.

The narratives of siblings provide a different perspective on the range of concerns that they face (Meyer, 2009). These stories indicate that siblings worry about their ability to live a normal life and whether, given their responsibilities to their brothers and sisters, it makes sense to have their own children. Some are concerned whether their siblings will ever enjoy their work or have a satisfying romantic relationship. Others wonder about societal responses if they choose not to maintain a close relationship with their sibling. Many report positive emotions regarding their siblings, some focus on the negative, and most have mixed feelings.

There are clear differences in the extent to which siblings are involved in the daily lives of their sisters and brothers. One brother who has twin siblings with developmental disabilities expressed the following view:

> No matter how much support I may one day provide, it won't be the same as the support Matt and Mike get from Mom and Dad. There is something different about being a sibling—a different perception. Maybe part of it is that we are not as protective; we are more willing to let our brothers and sisters take chances. Honestly, maybe part of it is that siblings are too busy with their own families and careers and just don't have the time to monitor their siblings. (Kramer, 2009, pp. 24–25[1])

---

[1]Passages in this chapter are from *Thicker Than Water: Essays by Adult Siblings of People With Disabilities* (pp. 24–120), edited by D. Meyer, 2009, Bethesda, MD: Woodbine House. Copyright 2009 by D. Meyer. Reprinted with permission.

In contrast, one sister of a young woman with multiple disabilities put it this way:

> I spend part of nearly every day doing something for Suzy. Her friends are now my friends. I quit working and now volunteer in my community on projects to support my sister, her nonprofit service providers, and our larger disability community. Some days I worry about losing myself, about becoming my sister's assistant instead of living my own life. And sometimes I get angry at my sister, especially on those days when I think she's being stubborn or selfish. On those days I feel that she has more power in our relationship. (S. Gray, 2009, p. 120)

The range of stories is impressive. Some siblings dramatically alter their lives and careers to spend time with their brothers and sisters whereas others, while acknowledging an attachment to their siblings, choose a more limited relationship. Whatever their differences, each of these siblings is attempting to balance a concern for his or her brothers and sisters with a need to attend to his or her own life and family.

In addition to displaying the diversity of sibling responses, these stories reveal the value of narrative in identifying individual experiences related to disability. In Chapter 9, I consider parent narratives and examine the narrative approach more fully.

9

LIFE CHALLENGES AND LIFE STORIES

I imagined a deliriously happy "empty nest" syndrome. Neither of us likes to travel, but sports are a big priority. I figured we would exercise, go to see the Rangers/Mavericks/Cowboys, etc., together. I envisioned weddings with lots of family pictures. There would be grandchildren to baby-sit. Life would be calm, easy, and sweet. (L. A. King & Raspin, 2004, p. 616)

People love stories, in books, movies, and other forms. Moreover, we construct stories of our own lives and share and revise them over time. By creating stories of our lives, we construct the salient features of our social identity, our sense of identity in relation to the important others in our lives. Our ability to construct stories that highlight the central features of our lives is an essential part of what it means to be a human being living in a social world.

This chapter considers the implications of research on narrative studies of lives for families touched by developmental disabilities. Narrative studies provide a useful complement to traditional psychological methods. Most psychological research, including most of the scholarship discussed in previous chapters, employs quantitative analysis of surveys and instruments devised by psychologists. In contrast, narrative studies employ an open-ended format in which the narrator supplies the structure and meaning. This form of study allows responders to raise questions not addressed by scales and surveys, issues that may be incorporated into future quantitative work.

http://dx.doi.org/10.1037/14192-009
Families of Children With Developmental Disabilities: Understanding Stress and Opportunities for Growth, by D. W. Carroll

I begin with an overview of the narrative approach, with an emphasis on the types of narrative themes found in lives with significant turning points or responses to unexpected events. Then I consider narratives of parents of children with disabilities, with an eye toward identifying common themes as well as the psychological impact of various narrative strategies. The chapter closes with some observations on the promise and limitations of narrative research on families of children with developmental disabilities.

THE NARRATIVE STUDY OF LIVES

Characteristics of Life Stories

To give us a point of reference when looking at narratives of parents of children with developmental disabilities, it will be useful to examine age-related changes in life narratives, particularly those in early and middle adulthood. In a series of publications, McAdams (2001, 2006, 2008) has explored the nature and function of personal narratives. A key concept in this work is *narrative identity*, which refers to a person's internalized, integrative, and evolving story of the self. People begin to form life narratives during adolescence and young adulthood, and these stories evolve throughout adulthood. The ways in which people make sense of their lives point to the common struggles in reconciling how we view ourselves internally versus how we present ourselves to others. McAdams (2008) suggested that it is through narrative identity that we come to terms with society.

McAdams (2008) identified six principles in the narrative study of lives: The self is storied, stories integrate lives, stories are told in social relationships, stories change over time, stories are cultural texts, and some stories are better than others. Humans are storytellers by nature, and stories are the best vehicle we have for conveying how humans intentionally strive for self-determined goals. Stories integrate lives by providing causal links between events at different points in time. Moreover, stories are intrinsically social, told by people to other people, and emphasize social connections and relationships. McAdams emphasized that stories are cultural texts in the sense that the themes that dominate stories vary with one's culture: Whereas Chinese narratives focus on how personal narratives may serve as guides for good social conduct, those of European Americans place a greater priority on self-expression.

Life Changes and Life Satisfaction

Two of the principles identified by McAdams (2008)—stories change over time and some stories are better than others—are particularly relevant for understanding lives in transition. Glück, Bluck, Baron, and McAdams (2005) explored changes in autobiographical narratives across adulthood. They were interested in the implicit theories of wisdom shown at adolescence, early midlife (30–40 years old), and older adulthood. The results were consistent with the bioecological approach to development (Bronfenbrenner & Ceci, 1994) in that the form of wisdom displayed by each group was in keeping with the life phase of the individual. Adolescents focused on empathy and support, early midlife adults on self-determination and assertion, and older adults on knowledge and flexibility.

L. A. King and Raspin (2004) explored narratives about life transitions. In particular, they examined how people relinquish previous expectations for their life story and develop new goals. In one study, divorced women who had been married for an average of 22 years wrote narrative descriptions of their best possible future selves before the divorce (retrospectively) as well as after the divorce. Participants also completed the Sentence Completion Test (Loevinger, 1985), a measure of ego development, and the Satisfaction With Life Scale (Diener, Emmons, Larson, & Griffin, 1985), a measure of subjective well-being. Independent raters scored the *salience* of the narratives (i.e., how easy it was to imagine) along with the degree of *elaboration* of the narratives (i.e., how much detail was provided).

L. A. King and Raspin (2004) found that the salience of the lost possible self was negatively correlated with the Satisfaction With Life Scale, whereas the salience of the current possible self was positively related to life satisfaction. Moreover, elaboration of the current possible self was positively associated with the Sentence Completion Test, and this relationship held in a follow-up analysis 2 years later. The authors concluded that positive well-being is predicted by a divestment of interest in "lost goals" accompanied by an investment in current life goals. L. A. King and Smith (2004) found similar results for gay men and lesbians who wrote about their straight (i.e., earlier) and gay possible selves. (For an example of writing in which the lost self was highly elaborated, see the quotation that began this chapter.)

These results suggest that some stories are better than others in the sense that they are more closely associated with subjective well-being, maturity, and life satisfaction. McAdams, Hoffman, Mansfield, and Day (1996) and McAdams (2001) distinguished between two types of growth themes: *agency* and *communion*. Agency themes emphasize the power, self-mastery, or achievement of the individual, whereas communion themes emphasize friendship, love, dialogue, and sharing. Bauer and McAdams (2004) found that people whose stories emphasized agentic growth were more likely to be satisfied with their life transitions, whereas those who emphasized communal growth were most likely to report higher levels of well-being in general (Bauer & McAdams, 2004). The type of transition also mattered. Themes of communal growth were more prevalent in those who changed religions but not those who changed careers. In addition, communion themes were positively correlated with satisfaction with life transitions for those who changed religions.

Redemption and Commitment

In addition to these general principles in adult narratives, researchers have identified themes that may be particularly significant for understanding disability experiences. Two of these themes are *redemption* and *commitment*. McAdams and Bowman (2001) and McAdams (2006) examined turning points in people's lives and redemption themes. Redemption occurs when an individual turns a negative life event into a more positive outcome. For example, the death of one's father might encourage a middle-aged man to reexamine his heavy commitment to work and rededicate himself to his family. McAdams and Bowman argued that redemption sequences are most commonly found in individuals with a high degree of *generativity*; that is, individuals wishing to contribute positively to the next generation.

McAdams, Diamond, de St. Aubin, and Mansfield (1997) analyzed the life stories of 40 highly generative and 30 less-generative adults. Highly generative adults were more likely to reconstruct the past and anticipate the future as variations on a prototypical commitment story in which the protagonist enjoys early family blessings, is sensitized to others' suffering at an early age, is guided by a clear and stable personal ideology, transforms or redeems bad scenes into good outcomes, and sets goals for the future to benefit society. Commitment stories sustain and reinforce the modern adult's efforts to contribute in positive ways to the next generation.

Redemption sequences may be contrasted with *contamination* sequences, in which emotionally positive events suddenly go bad—an emotionally positive experience is sullied or ruined by a bad outcome (McAdams, 2001; McAdams & Bowman, 2001). An example would be a protagonist who is proud at her graduation, until her father comments that she looked fat crossing the stage. For individuals whose life stories include a number of contamination sequences, the self does not grow; rather, the person stagnates or recycles through unsatisfying life plots. Contamination sequences are positively associated with depression and negatively associated with well-being. They are also more common in individuals who score low in generativity.

NARRATIVES OF PARENTS OF CHILDREN WITH DEVELOPMENTAL DISABILITIES

Several collections of narratives of families of children with developmental disabilities (Klein & Schive, 2001; Meyer, 1995, 2009; Soper, 2007) provide a rich supply of information about how parents and siblings of children with disabilities view their family life, their social world, and their future. Recently, researchers have undertaken qualitative analyses of these kinds of narratives. Here we begin by looking at five themes that have emerged from these analyses: stresses of the caregiver role, tensions with professionals, resilience and optimism, redemption, and the construction of meaning.

Stresses of the Caregiver Role

Many of the narratives emphasize the stresses associated with caring for a child with a disability. Myers, Mackintosh, and Goin-Kochel (2009) collected narratives from parents of children in the autistic spectrum via an online questionnaire. When asked how a child with autism has changed her life, one mother responded:

> I had to quit my job due to an inability to find child care. My younger kids imitate his behavior. Our house is very loud all the time people my son screams all the time! We have not gone on a date in over 2 years. (Myers et al., 2009, p. 673)

Another parent wrote of marital strain and the constant nature of the stress:

> My life is very closed, not a lot of people can deal with my son or are comfortable around him. I can't take him a lot of places because of crowds and noise, so we spend a lot of time at home or grandparents house. His biological father left when he was 3 and has contact maybe twice a year with his son. Has really limited a lot of things in our family. (Myers et al., 2009, p. 674)

Roll-Pettersson (2001) interviewed 46 parents of children with a cognitive disability. Some parents spoke of the stresses on their marriage; for example, one mother stated that

> I feel very locked up, my husband travels a lot . . . I'm not as free as I'd like to be. He is still like a little child, one is locked up with little children, but I'm still locked up, even though the children aren't little anymore. (Roll-Pettersson, 2001, p. 7)

Other parents emphasized the difficulties they have experienced in securing acceptance of their children in the wider society: "What I sometimes see, which is difficult, is that other children run away from her. She goes over to them to play, and they just look and then run away" (Roll-Pettersson, 2001, p. 7). Moreover, the social isolation experienced by children is prominent in their parents. Todd and Jones (2005) interviewed mothers of adolescents with intellectual disabilities, many of whom emphasized how their child's disability constricted their social life. One mother expressed the following sentiment:

> So I get out with my friends about once every two months. We go out in a gang. But I'm beginning to notice how different my life is from theirs. If I want to go out it's got to be really organized, they can do what they want . . . It just creeps up on you gradually that your life is really different . . . They're mostly working and go out whenever they fancy it. (Todd & Jones, 2005, pp. 396–397)

Tensions Between Parents and Professionals

Another major theme that emerged in these narratives was the tension that existed between parents and the medical and educational professionals who serve their children. Resch et al. (2010) conducted a qualitative study of the challenges experienced by parents of children with disabilities. Resch et al. (2010) identified four themes: lack of access to information and services, financial barriers, the struggle for school and community inclusion, and the need for family support. With regard to school and community inclusion, parents found the lack of support for inclusion frustrating. Efforts at inclusion were often impeded by what the parents perceived as low expectations:

> Many times, as parents, we'll go to an agency and the social worker sees the disability and she automatically labels our children. For them your child is not going to accomplish anything in life. Some people think that way and parents are confronted with those people. Unfortunately, it happens a lot of times. (Resch et al., 2010, p. 144)

In contrast, parents of children with disabilities had high expectations for their children:

> I have an eight year old that has Down Syndrome and now I am thinking college, you know . . . that's my issue now, because people say, "well kids that have special needs [are] not going to go to college," [but] they are [like everyone else] . . . they're not just on the other side and we try to make them part of the community." (Resch et al., 2010, p. 144)

Resch et al. (2010) noted that for some parents, the continual battle for inclusion led them to be labeled as troublemakers, adding a source of stress for parents who already felt excluded from their communities.

Other parents also emphasized differences with the professionals who served their children. One of the parents interviewed by Roll-Pettersson (2001) commented:

> I have met ones [psychologists] who wanted to put us into a certain model, the first one [referring to the question] with shock, etc. The same thing with the psychologist who places one in a certain theory that the psychologist has studied. I've experienced that rather often; they believe in a model and that's it. Even if it can go back and forth or vary, they don't believe it; no, you are placed in a model and that's it. (p. 8)

Similarly, one of the parents of children with autism spectrum disorder interviewed by Myers et al. (2009) commented:

> Public school has been a nightmare. We have had to fight for everything we've gotten for him. We have paid thousands of dollars for outside speech and psychological counseling, and tutoring which was not covered by insurance. I was called nearly every day by the school because of behavior issues. It drove us to the brink of emotional breakdown. (p. 676)

Myers et al. noted that some parents moved to a new city or state to receive the desired services for their children.

Optimism and Resilience

Several of the studies in which parents spoke of stresses and tensions also revealed evidence of optimism, resilience, and personal growth. One mother of a child with autism spectrum disorder studied by Myers et al. (2009) remarked on how her child changed her priorities:

> He has made us 'see the light' and reprioritize. Things we used to think were important are no longer important. Our goals are no longer career oriented. We enjoy life a little more. Our biggest priorities are being happy, having fun, and doing whatever it takes to make sure that E will be a self happy and sufficient adult. (p. 678)

Another parent from the same study expressed it this way:

> My son has so enriched my life that it is unbelievable. I have learned so much about living life fully, about God and the nature of man, about love. It hasn't been easy all the time, but I would not trade the experience for anything. I think regular kids are boring. You don't have to try to read their minds, expressions or mannerisms. I love him better than life itself. (Myers et al., 2009, p. 674)

Similarly, Retzlaff (2007) found that parents of children with Rett syndrome emphasized themes of resilience and coherence. Evidence of two types of resilience stories were found. In one, parents reported changes in family meanings very early in the interview; emphasized that their daughter had enriched their family life; and reported many examples of charming, enchanting moments with her. These parents focus on the person, not the disability. As one parent expressed it:

> We experience her so much as a gift. Her total being—we love her so much that we do not miss anything—on the contrary, we are grateful, that she has what she has. And we do not think about what she is missing. (Retzlaff, 2007, p. 252)

Other parents focus much more on the stresses and reported less social support. Retzlaff (2007) referred to the former stories as "stories of refound balance" and to the latter as "the long tedious walk uphill" (p. 252). Changes in family meaning played a less significant role for these families and occurred only after a long period of struggle.

Redemption

Some of the parent narratives evoked responses similar to the redemption theme identified by McAdams and colleagues (McAdams, 2001; McAdams & Bowman, 2001). For example, Fleischmann (2005) found that parents of children with autism sometimes created websites to help other parents:

> I have tried to include everything that I found useful: information on autism, diagnosis, treatments, health, nutrition and diets, conferences, sensory integration, applied behavior analysis, links and resources in the United States and especially Texas. Now I would like to pass on what I learned. I hope this will help you. (p. 309[1])

For some, the interest in helping others is a form of recognition of the help they received:

> When I discovered that my son S was autistic, I didn't know where to turn. I met another parent of an autistic child, who was able to point me in the right direction . . . So, this is my way of giving a little help to those who may be in need of it. (p. 309)

This mother, having received help from another parent in the past, now wishes to help others. The desire to help others can be characterized as a redemption theme, in the sense discussed by McAdams. By helping others, these parents are turning something initially bad into something good.

Other parents have found positive value for others in their experiences. One example is that when their children are included more in society, others benefit as well:

---

[1]Passages in this chapter are from "The Hero's Story and Autism: Grounded Theory Study of Websites for Parents of Children With Autism," by A. Fleischmann, 2005, *Autism*, 9, p. 309. Copyright 2005 by SAGE. Reprinted with permission.

> The biggest thing [my child] can contribute is to those other students in that school. They learn an understanding of kids who are different. [They learn] that kids who have special needs are not to be ignored or to be put in another building. You don't take them out of society—they're part of society. . . . So as much as he's learning socially from being in that classroom, those other kids are learning more. (G. King et al., 2009, p. 59)

For these parents, a positive outcome that emerges from their experience is that they can offer something positive to others. In the process, they feel a sense of belonging to a larger group.

Although some of these narratives resembled the redemption stories analyzed by McAdams and colleagues (McAdams, 2001; McAdams & Bowman, 2001), further research into the degree of similarity is warranted. It would be helpful, for example, to study parents to determine whether some of their early life experiences were similar to the observations that McAdams has made in terms of high levels of generativity (e.g., childhood advantages, awareness of others' suffering).

Construction of Meaning

Several lines of research highlight how parents construct meaning out of their experiences by changing core beliefs or revising their dreams for themselves or their children. These stories emphasize letting go of lost dreams along with constructing new possibilities for their children and themselves (Green, 2002; G. A. King, Zwaigenbaum, et al., 2006).

L. A. King and Patterson (2000) and L. A. King and Hicks (2006), using the methodology in a study discussed earlier in this chapter, examined how mothers of children with Down syndrome wrote about their best possible former and current selves. One mother described her former self in the following terms:

> Before I had my son, we were considering taking a job in California. I had visions of my blonde-haired son playing on the beach, being a movie star, or model. I also had planned on going back to work after a couple of months and continuing on with my career. I thought my son would ride his bike around the neighborhood with all his friends, play football, baseball, and all the other "boy" sports with the neighborhood children, effortlessly. I thought the developmental milestones would be attained, effortlessly. (L. A. King & Hicks, 2006, p. 130)

L. A. King and Patterson found results similar to those found in studies of divorced mothers and gay men and lesbians discussed earlier. The salience of current best possible self was related to subjective well-being in parents of children with Down syndrome. That is, investing in one's current goals (and divesting earlier ones) was positively correlated with a person's happiness.

In addition, L. A. King and Patterson (2000) found that elaboration of the lost possible self was associated with psychological growth. The mixture of acceptance of examination of former self and acceptance of current self emerges in the following narrative:

> I see myself on an exciting journey. I like who I am. I have many areas that need work but for the most part I'm present and attentive to my needs and dreams and goals. . . . I am finding that giving is truly more satisfying than receiving. I have had a challenge in accepting my son's DS. It's taken time but unconditional love and acceptance are truly there. . . . I want to work within the community to be an agent of change. We all have a time of being a caregiver—to our children or parents, or someone. I want to offer . . . tools for people to find their own balance and peace. . . . I am quite selfish by nature: My son has opened that perspective—a new window for loving and caring now exists for me. I'm proud that I have taken responsibility for my own growth and challenges. (L. A. King & Hicks, 2006, pp. 133–134)

L. A. King and Hicks noted that this participant demonstrated both a high level of self-knowledge and a level of self-deprecation often found in mature individuals. The ability to explicitly identify mistaken expectations appears to energize individuals to embark on new life paths.

Another way of finding meaning is through religion. Michie and Skinner (2010) examined narratives of mothers of children with fragile X syndrome. A majority of women interpreted their children's disabilities within a religious framework, viewing the disability less as a burden and more as a blessing and part of God's plan for their lives. Some of the mothers viewed the purpose in terms of some of their own characteristics:

> I feel that this is why God gave me Sara. I'm a stable person. I've always been a homebody. And, [God thought] "she'll be able to take care of a child with special needs." I think that's why He gave me her . . . I think there's always a reason behind everything. (Michie & Skinner, 2010, p. 107)

Interpreting their children's disability as a blessing did not occur immediately for these mothers, but rather over a period of time:

> It's so funny how the blessings come. Like now I feel like the luckiest person in the world to have been able to experience Danielle and how much joy she brings. But at the time that I'm sleep deprived and postpartum and breastfeeding and just, like, trying to get a shower in, the word "blessing" never at all came to mind. . . .Yeah, I do feel like religion plays a big part in helping you handle it or understand it, but not initially. It comes later. (Michie & Skinner, 2010, p. 99)

Although framing the experience of raising a child with a disability in religious terms did not eliminate the challenges associated with that experience, it provided a source of meaning for why a person's life is challenged in this way.

These reports attest to the ability of individuals to reframe their life stories in light of unexpected and difficult experiences. Consonant with research that suggests that positive affect contributes to the experience of meaning in life (L. A. King, Hicks, Krull, & Del Gaiso, 2006), these narratives suggest that such reframing may lead, in some instances, to a deeper, more satisfying life.

In summary, the narrative analyses discussed in this section both support and extend the research reviewed in previous chapters. The stories supplied by parents of children with disabilities included themes of stress, social isolation, professional skepticism, and optimism prevalent in studies that have primarily employed questionnaires and surveys. However, the narratives also extend previous research by revealing elements of redemption, redefinition, and meaning construction that have been less often emphasized in more traditional research formats. On the whole, the narratives provide a rich and well-rounded view of the experience of parenting a child with a disability.

Quantitative Analyses of Parental Narratives

Although most of the research on parental narratives has employed qualitative research methods, there have been a few efforts to examine these narratives quantitatively. Carroll (2008, 2009) analyzed narratives of parents of children with developmental disabilities using the Linguistic Inquiry and Word Count (LIWC) software developed by Pennebaker, Booth, and Francis (2007). The LIWC receives text files as input and produces measures of approximately 80 linguistic and psychological variables. Most measures are the percentages of various word types (e.g., pronouns, articles, emotion words) in the text. Previous studies have explored the relationships between LIWC measures and variables such as age, personality, and depression. For example, Stirman and Pennebaker (2001) compared poems written by writers who committed suicide with those of a group of poets matched in age and other variables. Suicidal poets used more first person singular pronouns than nonsuicidal poets, which is consistent with theories that posit that self-absorption is a contributing factor in suicide.

Carroll (2008) contrasted books written by parents of children with disabilities with books written by parents of healthy children. Books written by parents of children with developmental disabilities used fewer first person singular (I, my) and second-person pronouns (you, yours) but more first person plural (we, us) and third-person pronouns (he, she). In addition, parents of children with disabilities expressed more optimism (certainty, win) and less anger (fight, rage) than parents of healthy children. The results suggest that parents of children with disabilities wrote more about their children and others whereas parents of healthy children wrote more about themselves. This finding may indicate that parents of children with disabilities have immersed themselves so fully in their family's well-being that they have become less attentive to purely personal concerns. The study is consistent with research that identifies positive adjustments to the challenges of parenting a child with developmental disabilities.

A subsequent study (Carroll, 2009) examined the effect of diagnostic uncertainty on narratives of parents with developmental disorders by comparing narratives of parents of children with Down syndrome with narratives of parents of children with other developmental disabilities. The latter group included children with less clear diagnoses such as autism and cerebral palsy, as well as some disabilities that were not clearly diagnosed. Parents of children with Down syndrome made fewer references to tentativeness (*maybe, perhaps*), insight (*know, think*), causation (*because, conclude*), and sadness (*cry, grief*) than did parents of children with other developmental disabilities, suggesting that diagnostic uncertainty may increase both cognitive processing and negative emotions in parents of children with developmental disabilities.

Carroll (2009) also connected these parental narratives to some themes discussed in the work of McAdams and colleagues (McAdams, 2001; McAdams & Bowman, 2001). The notion of redemption sequences, in which individuals are able to turn negative life events into positive outcomes, appeared to be more common in parents of children with Down syndrome, who tended to view their lives as transformed in positive ways. Although redemption themes were also found in parents of children with other developmental disabilities, the latter narratives were tinged with elements of sadness.

Psychological Consequences of Narrative Strategies

What consequences do these stories have for the parents? Is there a relationship between the kinds of stories they share and their psychological well-being? There is reason to think that this is the case. A number of studies have examined the effects of writing on physical and psychological health. The process of writing one's story can have a powerful effect on physical health as measured by visits to physician offices. Moreover, certain types of writing seem to be particularly helpful. Pennebaker, Mehl, and Niederhoffer (2003) found that stories that express high levels of positive emotion, moderate levels of negative emotion, and high levels of cognitive processing were predictive of better physical health (e.g., fewer physician visits). In other words, when people write about stressful or difficult events and acknowledge some of the frustrations they have experienced but are nonetheless able to ultimately emphasize more positive outcomes, they tend to be physically healthier.

L. A. King, Scollon, Ramsey, and Williams (2000) examined subjective well-being and ego development in the narratives of parents of children with Down syndrome. A sample of 87 parents of children with Down syndrome wrote narratives about learning that their child had Down syndrome. They also completed questionnaire measures of subjective well-being and a test of ego development. A subgroup of 42 individuals participated in a follow-up study 2 years later. Parents who recounted their stories with happy endings showed greater subjective well-being at both times. But that is not all. L. A. King et al. (2000) found that parents who expressed a sense of struggle and accommodation to meet their child's needs but still ended their narratives on a positive note displayed the greatest level of ego development, or psychological maturity. In contrast, thinking about previously cherished "lost possible selves" was associated with higher levels of distress.

Limitations and Future Prospects

At the present time, the narrative study of parents of children with disabilities is in its infancy. The narratives that exist paint a vivid portrait of the life of parents of children with disabilities. Confidence increases in the centrality of a theme when it emerges not only in response to the questions posed by researchers but also in the more open-ended interview formats preferred by narrative researchers.

The most significant limitation of the existing studies is that most are descriptive in nature. However compelling these stories are, questions of validity linger until researchers can find meaningful relationships between narrative themes and more standard psychological measures of well-being, life satisfaction, and happiness. In this respect, the studies of McAdams and colleagues provide a model for disability researchers to emulate.

The narrative study of lives touched by disabilities can, in turn, illuminate some of the less-studied regions of narrative studies. Individuals with disabilities and their families have a wealth of nonnormative experiences that figure into their life stories in rich and complicated ways. These narratives may extend earlier studies of lives in transition in productive ways. For example, it might be interesting to compare the time frames associated with divesting oneself of earlier life goals for individuals going through a divorce relative to parents raising a child with a disability. Surely, extending narrative analyses to families touched by disability will profit both fields.

One of the salient findings of the narrative approach is that when our experiences violate our expectations, individuals seek out ways to make sense of the discrepant event. Although there is evidence that parents of children with disabilities construct meaning in a number of ways, such meaning making is not always necessary or even always beneficial. In fact, current research suggests that the relationship between meaning and adjustment is complex and that some forms of meaning making are more closely related to well-being than others (C. L. Park, 2010). The extent to which making sense promotes well-being is a key component of understanding the processes of bereavement, which is the topic of Chapter 10.

10

DEATH AND BEREAVEMENT

The attitude of people seems to be "life must go on" or "life will go on." There is an ignorance of the fact that Carole was my life. I spent the vast majority of her waking hours each day trying to make life better for her. So how could life go on? (Todd, 2007, p. 642)

Individuals with developmental disabilities often have a shorter life expectancy than do those without disabilities. The extent of the diminished expectancy is related to both the severity and the type of disability. It is not uncommon for individuals with severe cerebral palsy to have a life span of less than 20 years (R. T. Katz, 2003), and individuals with profound intellectual disability have a significantly lower life expectancy than that of the general population (Patja, Iivanainen, Vesala, Oksanen, & Ruoppila, 2000). Although life expectancies for individuals with developmental disabilities have increased dramatically over the past few decades, persons with Down syndrome continue to have a heightened risk of death from congenital heart defects (Yang, Rasmussen, & Friedman, 2002). On the whole, the experience of losing a child remains more common for parents of children with disabilities than for parents of typically developing children.

http://dx.doi.org/10.1037/14192-010
Families of Children With Developmental Disabilities: Understanding Stress and Opportunities for Growth,
by D. W. Carroll

A growing scientific literature is now available that attests to the variability of grief reactions. Some of the newer research has encouraged psychologists to revisit older assumptions, including the view that prolonged and difficult "grief work" is necessary for adjustment to loss. Recent work suggests that bereaved individuals may display a range of reactions. In particular, it has become apparent that some individuals maintain a sense of psychological well-being despite their losses.

In contrast to the burgeoning literature on bereavement in general, research on parental responses to the death of a child with developmental disabilities is sparse. However, we can learn from individuals who share some features with these parents, including individuals who care for the elderly and parents who have experienced the sudden death of a typically developing child (e.g., in a motor vehicle accident). In the former case, much of a person's life may be wrapped up in the care given to another person over a long period of time, thus making the person's death a challenge to the caregiver's identity. In the latter case, parents whose children die face a nonnormative experience that may be difficult for family and friends to appreciate fully and respond to.

This chapter begins by discussing traditional and more contemporary psychological theories of bereavement. Then I turn to the narratives of parents whose child with a disability has died and identify some common themes. The final section explores whether some parents of children with disabilities experience positive psychological growth following their child's death.

PSYCHOLOGICAL STUDIES OF BEREAVEMENT

Traditional Views of Bereavement

Psychological theories about how people respond to losses of loved ones tend to focus on the grief and emotional distress that the individuals experience. In part, this is because much of the knowledge about bereavement has come from individuals who have sought professional treatment for their grief (Bonanno, 2004). Many psychologists and therapists have concluded that these responses are typical or perhaps even necessary for individuals who have suffered losses to return to mental health. In a seminal article, Wortman and Silver (1989) challenged this conclusion. Specifically, Wortman and Silver (1989) addressed the expectations that depression is inevitable following loss, that distress is a necessary part of bereavement, that failure to experience distress is a sign of pathology, that it is necessary for a person to "work through" or process a loss, and that recovery or resolution occurs following a loss. The authors concluded that the available empirical research failed to support and in some cases contradicted these assertions.

Wortman and Silver (2001) revisited these issues. As in the earlier study, most of the research focuses on the loss of a spouse, but newer studies have examined the loss of a child or parent. They found that 20% to 35% of people experience depression following the loss of a spouse, depending on the sample and the assessment procedures. Although some critics have charged that some individuals may be experiencing "absent grief," such a notion is difficult to assess. Some people experience a sense of relief at a loss, if their experience prior to the loss involved a high level of distress (Wheaton, 1990). In their earlier paper, Wortman and Silver (1989) were not able to identify any research supporting the concept of "working through" a loss. More recently, such studies have been done but do not provide much support for the concept. For example, Nolen-Hoeksema, McBride, and Larson (1997) found that recently bereaved men who ruminated more about their losses showed more evidence of depression over the following year. In short, the earlier paper found little empirical research directly pertaining to the key assumptions of the traditional "grief work" hypothesis, whereas the later paper reviewed an increasing number of studies that found little support for the hypothesis.

A related question concerns the extent to which individuals who have experienced sudden, traumatic loss search for meaning in their lives. C. G. Davis, Wortman, Lehman, and Silver (2000) studied 124 parents coping with the death of their infant from sudden infant death syndrome and 93 adults coping with the loss of their spouse or child in a motor vehicle accident. The researchers asked the participants whether they had ever searched for meaning following their loss. Results indicated that a significant subset of individuals did not search for meaning, yet these individuals scored higher on measures of adjustment than those who did. Those who did find meaning, although better adjusted than those who searched for and did not find meaning, did not move on. Rather, they continued to pursue the issue of meaning fervently.

Such results have implications for grief therapy. Neimeyer (2000) conducted a meta-analysis of studies that randomly assigned individuals to different grief treatments and found that the tangible benefit of treatment was small. Moreover, the studies also revealed evidence that some individuals have worse psychological health after grief therapy than before. Neimeyer suggested that the notion of searching for meaning that guides some treatment programs may be too limited and that a richer, more inclusive notion of bereavement may be necessary to provide a stronger basis for clinical intervention.

Different Patterns of Bereavement

Recent studies underscore the multifaceted and variable nature of bereavement. Although the search for meaning may be an important part of the bereavement process for some individuals, it is not universal, nor is its absence a sign of pathology. Bonanno (2004) argued that traditional approaches to bereavement do not place sufficient attention on the capacity of individuals to thrive after extremely aversive events. Bonanno suggested that resilience is a distinct trajectory from the process of recovery, that resilience is more common than is often believed, and that there are many pathways to resilience.

Bonanno et al. (2002) gathered prospective data on more than 200 individuals several years before the death of their spouse and at 6 and 18 months postloss. The authors identified several bereavement patterns, including *common grief* (defined as heightened distress at the time of loss, followed by recovery), *chronic grief* (distress before, during, and after loss), and *resilience* (higher levels of positive affect throughout the bereavement process). They found that common and chronic grief patterns were relatively infrequent (10.7% and 15.6% of the sample, respectively) and that resilience was the most common pattern (45.9%). The resilient individuals had low levels of depression, both before and 18 months after their loss. Before bereavement, the resilient group did not report difficulties in their marriage, but they did have relatively high scores on measures (e.g., acceptance of death, emotional stability) that suggested an ability to adapt well to loss. Resilient individuals also tended to have high levels of instrumental support (e.g., financial support, help with the home). Similar results were found in a study of bereaved spouses, parents, and caregivers of a chronically ill life partner (Bonanno, Moskowitz, Papa, & Folkman, 2005). Half of each sample showed the resilience pattern, and close friends rated the resilient individuals as more positive and better adjusted than individuals showing other bereavement patterns.

Research by Bauer and Bonanno (2001) connected studies of bereavement with the life-story model of identity discussed in the previous chapter. As we have seen, McAdams (2001) suggested that people construct life stories that emphasize continuity. Bauer and Bonanno interviewed individuals whose spouses died. These individuals faced considerable discontinuity in their life roles following their loss. The authors suggested that the interviewees transformed their discontinuity into continuity by realizing how the personal meanings of activities before the loss can continue, perhaps in modified form, in new activities. For example, although the spouse's death made going to the ocean with the spouse impossible, it was still possible to go alone and to share the experience with others who also enjoyed the ocean alone. The types of transformations suggested by Bauer and Bonanno, however, are to be distinguished from the notion of "grief work" in that the transformational process need not be either prolonged or painful.

Factors Associated With Favorable Adjustment

As already noted, some factors (e.g., acceptance of death) are associated with more favorable adjustment following loss of a loved one. *Expressive flexibility*, which is defined as the ability to modulate emotional expressions in relation to situational demands, is also associated with favorable adjustment following loss. Bonanno, Papa, Lalande, Westphal, and Coifman (2004) found that the ability to enhance and suppress emotional expression predicted long-term adjustment among New York City college students in the aftermath of the September 11 attacks. Students participated in a laboratory task in which they tried to enhance or suppress emotional expression or behave normally on a series of trials. In this study, students' expressive flexibility predicted adjustment over their first 2 years of college. In addition, deficits in expressive flexibility have been associated with grief patterns in which individuals have strong yearnings for the deceased loved one, disbelief at the loss, and a pervasive sense that life is meaningless (Gupta & Bonanno, 2011). Deficits in expressive flexibility may hinder adjustment by making it more difficult for individuals to oscillate between periods of deep sadness, in which they share painful feelings with others, and periods in which feelings are suppressed to attend to the demands of daily activities.

Pennebaker, Mayne, and Francis (1997) examined linguistic predictors of adaptive bereavement in a set of studies. In one study, Pennebaker et al. (2007) explored whether the words that people used in disclosing a personal trauma would predict improvements in psychological and physical health. Words associated with insight (e.g., *realize, understand, consider*) and causation (e.g., *cause, effect, because*) were linked to improvements in physical but not mental health. A high proportion of positive words was associated with better health, but no evidence suggested that expressing negative emotions was beneficial to a person's health. In the second study, the researchers found that word usage in interviews with men who had lost their partners due to AIDS predicted mental health 1 year later. These results suggest that "processing" a loss may be adaptive, but in a context that focuses on positive emotions more than negative emotions.

BEREAVEMENT IN PARENTS OF A CHILD WITH A DISABILITY

As already noted, the literature on bereavement in parents of children with developmental disabilities is limited. Reilly, Hastings, Vaughan, and Huws (2008) suggested that we might gain insight into these parents' experiences by examining related cases, including parental bereavement outside of disabilities. Reilly, Hastings, et al. found gender differences in parental grief following a child's death from cancer, with mothers reporting more intense and longer grief reactions than did fathers. When a child's death was sudden, grief was more pronounced. At least some parents continue to experience depressive symptoms many years after their child's death (Rogers, Floyd, Seltzer, Greenberg, & Hong, 2008). Part of the reason may be the social constraints on discussing an infant's death, which have been linked to depressive symptoms in bereaved mothers (Lepore, Silver, Wortman, & Wayment, 1996). Lepore et al. (1996) found that a measure of social constraints (e.g., how often bereaved parents felt they had to keep their feelings to themselves because they made others uncomfortable) predicted depression symptoms in mothers. For socially constrained mothers, the number of intrusive thoughts 3 weeks after the infant's death was positively correlated with depressive symptoms 18 months later.

Similarly, some clues may be found in studies of individuals who served as long-term caregivers, often for elderly family members. Boerner, Schulz, and Horowitz (2004) studied 217 individuals who cared for a family member with dementia and found evidence for both positive and negative responses. Caregivers who reported higher levels of benefit associated with caregiving also reported more depression and grief following the death of the family member. Robinson-Whelen, Tada, MacCallum, McGuire, and Kielcot-Glaser (2001) found that the consequences of long-term caregiving endure long after the caregiving itself has ceased. Although former caregivers experienced decreases in stress, their levels of depression and loneliness took as long as 3 years to recover to the level of noncaregivers.

It is likely that the patterns of bereavement in families touched by disability are similar in some respects to other cases but contain some unique elements. We may begin by examining existing studies for common themes. Four of these themes are sudden or unexpected death, the physical nature of loss, double transition, and disenfranchised grief.

Sudden or Unexpected Death

One common theme in interviews with parents was that the death of their child was often perceived as sudden or unexpected. This may seem surprising, given the child's disabilities. However, even though parents are often informed that their child may have a shortened life span, estimates of life expectancy are typically inexact.

Todd (2007) interviewed 13 parents on the deaths of their children with intellectual disabilities. Several parents commented that their child's death came in a sudden and unexpected manner. One parent commented that

> I once asked a neurologist when Marie was three about her life expectancy. I wanted to make the best of whatever time I had. He did say "Well the nature of these children, it isn't likely that she'll attain adulthood." So we went straight out and bought a video camera. Everyone expected her to be an ill child but she wasn't at all. She never had any illnesses of note. (Todd, 2007, p. 640)

Mothers and fathers sometimes differ in their perceptions of the suddenness of the child's death. Reilly, Huws, Hastings, and Vaughan (2008) conducted semistructured interviews with nine mothers whose children with intellectual disabilities had died. Mothers understood and prepared for the loss of their child more than fathers did. One mother put it this way:

> I always knew that it would happen, and my husband never did. He . . . Once she'd come out of hospital he sort of thought, um, that they'd got it all wrong and that she would just be okay. . . . I always knew that this would happen, and I kind of always knew that that would be the way that I would find her one day. (D. Reilly, Huws, et al., 2008, p. 550)

Some parents express a profound sense of loss if they were not present at the time of their child's death. Milo (1997) interviewed mothers about the life and death of their children with developmental disabilities. One mother not present at her child's death shared the following:

> I feel like I was robbed of something very important. I wasn't able to say goodbye. I think it would have been so much easier if I could have, if they had called me. . . . It still hurts. It hurt a lot. Because I feel like I was just robbed of that closure. (Milo, 1997, p. 466)

These parents often expressed considerable distress over the fact that they had not had an opportunity to say goodbye to their children.

Physical Nature of Loss

Another theme is that the loss these parents experience is not only emotional but also physical. For many parents, caring for a disabled child is a physically intimate experience. As a consequence, the loss is felt in physical terms:

> It was a physical loss! It really was! It was surprising how physical it felt. Physical in my body, physical in my arms. I've two other children and holding them was nothing like holding Marie. You were always lifting, always carrying, always holding. There were lots of cuddles. (Todd, 2007, p. 642)

Davies (2005) conducted a qualitative study of mothers of children with cerebral palsy and noted that it was important for these mothers to spend time with their child's body after death. The mothers who were interviewed planned to have their child's body cared for at the children's hospice rather than in a mortuary or funeral home so that they could visit their child at any time. This arrangement provided them the privacy to hold their child and to place the body in the coffin. Similarly, in Todd's (2007) study, one parent described the difficulty in letting go:

> Then the police arrived because it was an unexpected death. The dreadful thing was thinking how to give them back our child. I remember saying "I don't know when to let go!" I didn't know whether to hold her for a few minutes more. You're holding her and she literally looked asleep, like every other time I had held her but I was looking for any movement. I was in the room for three hours. And then you walk away and walk out and it's such a gorgeous day! And all this has happened to you. (pp. 641–642)

Double Transition

Milo's (1997) study of maternal bereavement suggested that mothers experienced a double transition when their child with a disability died. Unlike mothers of typically developing children who die in a sudden accident, these mothers were faced with two profoundly significant life experiences in succession. First, they tried to make sense of their life with a child with a disability, then their life without that child. One mother whose child with cerebral palsy died at the age of 7 said:

> After I lost Annie I was back to square one. Well, she's gone now so who am I? Am I still that person? Who, who am I? I was very lonely and lost, lost, lost. I said, "What am I going to do now?" (Milo, 1997, p. 456)

These mothers created a life story in which their role as a caregiver was central. Thus, when their children died, they needed to reevaluate and revise that life story.

In a study of fathers' bereavement, Wood and Milo (2001) found that fathers also expressed a double sense of loss:

> It took me six years finally before I said, "Gee this is stupid, let Katie be Katie, let me just enjoy her as her dad rather than try to be her therapist, her teacher and stuff. She is going to be this way and accept her." I had just gotten there and she died. (p. 645)

Other fathers expressed a sense of bewilderment over the sudden loss of their role as father of a child with a disability. With the change came a complicated mix of relief and guilt:

Even to this day I can't believe it. I don't have to change diapers any more. I don't have to worry about her any more. I don't have to plan things in advance. I am free now. That still makes me feel a little guilty. (Wood & Milo, 2001, p. 645)

Disenfranchised Grief

A major theme that recurs in many of these narratives is that parents who have lost a child with a developmental disability often did not receive social validation of their loss. Other people often failed to appreciate the nature of their loss, were unwilling to converse about it, or both. As a consequence, parents often felt isolated and unsupported. These experiences appear to be an example of *disenfranchised grief*, which is a form of grief that occurs when an individual experiences a loss that is not publicly acknowledged or openly mourned (Doka & Lavin, 2003). Examples may include perinatal death, death from HIV/AIDS, and cases in which the relationship to the deceased cannot be acknowledged. Attig (2004) suggested that recovery from loss begins when it is socially recognized. If so, the process is inevitably more complicated when a child with a disability dies.

Todd (2007) suggested that when children with disabilities die, their parents experience something similar, which he referred to as *silenced grief*. These parents often felt that family members and friends did not easily recognize the depth and scale of their loss. One person commented: "I don't think members of my family understood. You know a cousin said 'Well this time for you to start living!' They didn't know anything. And they saw Frances as a burden. If only they knew" (Todd, 2007, p. 644). Several of the mothers in the study by D. Reilly, Huws, et al. (2008), discussed earlier, also felt that their loss was undervalued by others because the child had an intellectual disability:

I remember when Simon died somebody actually said to Martin well it's not like losing your own. And you know, the other thing they say about children with disabilities is it was a blessed release wasn't it. And I want to go hang on. This was their life . . . this shows what you know about our children. (D. Reilly, Huws, et al., 2008, p. 551)

As in the Lepore et al. (1996) study discussed earlier, social constraints often play a role in limiting the social support to parents during bereavement. Friends and family members may say something inappropriate or perhaps say nothing at all for fear of saying the wrong thing.

Schormans (2004) examined the experience of losing a child with a developmental disability from the perspective of foster parents in the child welfare system. Foster parents thought of themselves as parents and experienced losses comparable with those of birth parents. Like birth parents, their identification as legitimate grievers was often not recognized by family and friends, who referred to their children as "only foster kids." The significance of their loss, however, was recognized by child welfare agencies, for at least some of the foster parents.

The result of this disenfranchisement is that the connection between parents and the larger social circle, never strong for many parents, is particularly weak at their time of grief. Adding to their social isolation is the conduct of some of the professionals who provided services for their children who, the parents believed, withdrew with too must haste. In one instance, parents were told on the day of the child's funeral that social services would not be seeing them anymore (Todd, 2007). The withdrawal of support was not unexpected by some but was seen as indicative of a longer period of dissatisfaction with service intervention during the child's lifetime (Todd & Jones, 2003). The withdrawal of services exacerbated a profound sense of social isolation in some parents:

> You feel really, really isolated because the circles that you've been moving in with like the hospices, doctors, the nurses, school . . . it's like your whole world has collapsed. It's not just Jake you've lost; it's all of that as well. (D. Reilly, Huws, et al., 2008, p. 551)

A recent study by Runswick-Cole (2010) discussed the death of children with disabilities from a sociological perspective. The author suggested that just as parents have difficulties in obtaining appropriate support services during their child's life, it is challenging for parents to receive appropriate services during the bereavement process. One parent commented, "No one wants to talk about the death of a child, and that is why there are no services for families like mine" (Runswick-Cole, 2010, p. 814). Runswick-Cole highlighted the social isolation and poverty that parents experienced following the loss of their child.

Additional research on the similarities and differences among parents who have lost a child with a disability and other groups is warranted, but some preliminary conclusions are in order. The experience of parents who have lost a child with a disability appears both to resemble and differ from the experiences of other caregivers. Caregiving is often a full-time job and the death of the person needing care may constitute a challenge to caregivers' sense of identity, but the nonnormative experience of losing a child may isolate parents more than is the case for caregivers of elderly individuals. In addition, parents who have lost a child with a disability have some overlap with parents who have lost a typically developing child, but differences can be seen. Both may experience a sudden loss, but the double transitions that parents of disabled children often experience as well as the physical nature of the loss may be less common in parents of typically developing children.

POSTTRAUMATIC GROWTH FOLLOWING THE DEATH OF A CHILD WITH A DISABILITY

To this point, the discussion has focused on the stress associated with the death of a child with a disability, including stressors associated with grief generally as well as stressors more specific to this situation. However, some research studies suggest that parents experience personal growth following their child's death. These studies present a point of view slightly different from those, cited earlier in the chapter, that have found individuals to be resilient in the face of the death of a loved one. In contrast, some parents of children with developmental disabilities experience significant distress or even trauma, but also positive growth following the death of their child.

Positive Outcomes Following the Loss of a Loved One

Frantz, Farrell, and Trolley (2001) identified some of the positive outcomes that may occur following death: social bonds may be strengthened or newly established, sense of spirituality may be increased, beliefs and lifestyle may be changed, and emotionality (including humor) may be increased. The authors interviewed 397 adults whose loved ones had died approximately 1 year earlier. Most respondents believed that they had learned something from the experience (98%), that something positive had come out of the experience (84%), and that they had changed in some way (85%).

Similarly, Tedeschi and Calhoun (2004) suggested that posttraumatic growth occurs in a significant minority or even a majority of people who have experienced a significant loss. The growth may be seen in terms of more meaningful personal relationships, changed priorities, spiritual growth, or an increased appreciation for life in general. The authors cautioned about individual differences in this area, and noted that gender, personality, and other variables may influence a person's response to a traumatic loss.

Positive Outcomes Following the Loss of a Child With a Disability

Although no studies have specifically investigated positive parental responses to the death of a child with developmental disabilities, some of the reports cited earlier highlighted positive outcomes, albeit ones mixed with negative outcomes in a complicated way. An example is Milo's (1997) study of mothers' responses to the life and death of a child with a developmental disability. Milo reported that when the mothers she interviewed tallied up the joys and sorrows, seven of the eight believed that parenting and losing a child with a developmental disability was an experience they would never give up. Milo commented that parents were well aware of the paradox of something both difficult and valuable, as suggested by the following quote:

> I used to wish that she would die. I remember before I brought her home from the hospital thinking, God, I wish she would just die and then I wouldn't have to bring her home and go through this and put the kids through this. And I just couldn't have been more wrong. (Milo, 1997, p. 457)

Another parent expressed it this way:

> If I were pregnant and knew the child were handicapped, I would not bring that child into this world . . . and for me that is not a conflict. I would not put a child through that and I would not put myself through that . . . it's extremely painful. But having said that, I can't say I really regret it either, my life, or Brian. Brian brought me so much, brought everyone around him so much, so I don't know. It sounds like a contradiction, but to me it's not. (Milo, 1997, p. 457)

Once again, the mixture of positive and negative emotions is prominent in ways that may be difficult for others to appreciate fully.

Some of the mothers interviewed by Milo (1997) also found the life and death of their children as something that led to personal growth. For some, the growth came in the form of developing assertiveness in the service of their child:

> Annie made me who I am today. She gave me the strength to stand up for myself and to realize the power I have as a person. I never had that before. I was not vocal, I was young, I was just married and in la-la land. I never actually understood who I was as a person, and Annie made me grow. (Milo, 1997, p. 459)

For others, the focus was on a sense of priorities:

> I didn't even know what priorities were prior to her being. It just has made me so in tune to every aspect of humanity. Not just to say people of different colors and even different cultural experiences and different economics. Now I can really look at the world, I think, from clearer eyes, and be more sensitive to everybody. You look at people for who they really are. (Milo, 1997, pp. 459–460)

For still others, there was a spiritual dimension:

> When I see what I went through, what other people go through I don't understand the reason why the child suffers and the parent agonizes . . . it

amazes me that you can love so much and then it's taken away, it's kinda harsh. . . . I almost thought of giving up the faith, but it was all too real. . . . God was all I had and I came to realize that God was all I really needed. (Milo, 1997, p. 460)

Many of the mothers found meaning and benefit in the life and death of their children and were able to continue to see the world as a benevolent and purposeful place.

Similar sentiments emerged in a study of six parents whose child with Down syndrome died of a congenital heart condition (D. Reilly, Huws, Hastings, & Vaughan, 2010). Some parents commented that they had grown stronger through the experience:

I perhaps have realised that I am a stronger . . . there's like an inner strength that rises up and you do, as I say, you find it within you to cope with these things. And so I guess I look back and I think, gosh, you know, we have been through a lot and we have come out the other side, you know. (D. Reilly et al., 2010, p. 410)

Others indicated that the life and death of their child caused the parent to reflect on priorities:

It's not something that wouldn't affect anything. So yes it affected us for all the good and all the better or all the worse. I don't think it changed it probably. It changed both of us the way we think of each other and think of life and things I suppose. I mean I became much less driven by work after that. The only thing that matters now is [my wife and daughter]. (D. Reilly et al., 2010, pp. 410–411)

D. Reilly et al. (2010) reported that all of the parents they interviewed shared at least some positive reflections on their experience. The mixture of emotions that death may bring, while challenging for outsiders to appreciate fully, may actually connect couples closer together.

In their review of the literature on parental bereavement following the death of a child with intellectual disabilities, D. E. Reilly, Hastings, et al. (2008) identified some areas for future research. One was the role of ethnicity in parental caregiving and bereavement. Parents from different racial or ethnic backgrounds may draw on different resources and cultural beliefs (including religious beliefs), which are likely to influence the course of grief and bereavement. In addition, although some studies suggest gender differences in bereavement, few concrete differences have been found. This topic deserves further study.

Although the studies to date suggest that parents often find benefits from the life and death of a child with a developmental disability, they do not provide a full account of the positive character strengths that may emerge from this experience. In fairness, the studies were not intended to do so. Research on posttraumatic growth that is more directly based on the positive psychology framework may hold much value. Many of the character strengths identified by positive psychologists (N. Park, Peterson, & Seligman, 2006)— such as courage, spirituality, and gratitude—appear to be good candidates for examination.

A fuller account of the grief and bereavement process should be of significant value to service providers. Although there is considerable variability in parental responses, there are common themes that are not likely to be obvious to those who have not been a parent of a child with disabilities.

11

CLINICAL IMPLICATIONS

You know what it is, it's a lifestyle of behavior modification. Everything in your daily life, everything you do, is behavior modification. How is this going to affect [my child]? The way you speak to him, the schedules—ignore the negative, reinforce the positive. And the whole—our entire life, seven days a week—is that. (G. King, Baxter, Rosenbaum, Zwaigenbaum, & Bates, 2009, p. 59[1])

As the previous chapters attest, the journey of families of children with developmental disabilities can be emotionally complex. Parents may grieve the loss of the child they expected and experience frustration and challenges in securing appropriate services for their children. However, they may also discover that their child with a disability brings joy and perhaps even a spiritual dimension to their lives. Siblings sometimes resent the parental attention that their disabled siblings require, but as they mature it is not uncommon for them to be proud of their siblings, and they sometimes willingly take on added responsibilities in caring and advocating for them.

The mixture of emotions present in these families leads them down different paths. Some families, much like the resilient individuals prominent in the bereavement literature, thrive despite the obvious challenges

---

[1]From "Belief Systems of Families of Children With Autism Spectrum Disorders or Down Syndrome," by G. King, D. Baxter, P. Rosenbaum, L. Zwaigenbaum, and A. Bates, 2009, *Focus on Autism and Other Developmental Disabilities*, 24, p. 59. Copyright 2009 by SAGE. Reprinted with permission.

http://dx.doi.org/10.1037/14192-011
Families of Children With Developmental Disabilities: Understanding Stress and Opportunities for Growth, by D. W. Carroll

they face. Other families are largely successful in adapting to a child with unexpected needs but benefit from the informal social support groups discussed in Chapter 5. Still others have more significant emotional needs and seek professional help, which is the focus of this chapter.

I first consider guidelines for psychologists in dealing with individuals with disabilities and their families. Then I discuss the efficacy of two forms of clinical intervention with families of children with developmental disorders: programs designed to reduce stress in families and interventions based on positive psychology principles that seek to go beyond alleviating suffering and focus on the promotion of engagement and meaning.

GUIDELINES FOR ASSESSMENT AND INTERVENTION WITH PERSONS WITH DISABILITIES

Recently, the American Psychological Association (APA) published guidelines to assist psychologists to "conceptualize and implement more effective, fair, and ethical psychological assessments and interventions with persons with disabilities" (APA, 2012, p. 43). The 22 guidelines provide recommendations with regard to disability awareness, assessment, and interventions. Although most of the guidelines deal with individuals with disabilities, some attention is given to family issues. Psychologists are encouraged to recognize that families of individuals with disabilities possess strengths as well as challenges and that many families are resilient and regard their experiences related to disability in terms of meaningful growth.

The guidelines are meant to remedy a lack of attention to disability issues in many graduate programs in clinical psychology. Olkin (2002) looked at the frequency of disability courses in APA-accredited clinical programs in 1989 (1 year before the passage of the Americans With Disabilities Act) and in 1999. The percentage of programs without any disability courses actually increased from 1989 (76%) to 1999 (89%). The modal number of required courses on disability in 1999 was still zero, as it had been in 1989 (Olkin & Pledger, 2003). Moreover, much of the curricular attention was devoted to the medical model; only seven out of 210 programs had a course on the psychosocial aspects of disability (Olkin & Pledger, 2003). Olkin noted that graduate coursework on disability issues, because of its paucity, does not adequately prepare students to deal with clients with disabilities. In addition, such limited curricula might lead graduate students with disabilities to feel marginalized.

The lack of graduate training in disabilities has been shown to be a significant obstacle in providing effective services to clients with disabilities. Leigh, Powers, Vash, and Nettles (2004) surveyed psychologists who were APA members to determine perceptions of barriers to providing services, support needs, and factors related to successful treatment. Of the 481 respondents, 176 reported having a disability. Of respondents with disabilities, 22% reported that lack of expertise was a barrier that hindered providing services to clients with disabilities; the corresponding percentage for respondents without disabilities was 11%. Psychologists with disabilities were also more likely to identify support needs such as additional training or information about disability services. Both groups of respondents indicated that having a personal connection to people with disabilities promoted successful interventions, but the percentage was higher for respondents with disabilities (61%) than for respondents without disabilities (43%). The authors recommended additional training for psychologists on disability issues, and they suggested that psychologists with disabilities could be an important resource.

It is too early to tell whether the new guidelines will spur additional curricular efforts related to disability issues in clinical doctoral programs. A portion of such a curriculum would concern interventions that have proven to be effective for families of children with developmental disabilities, the issue to which I now turn.

INTERVENTION PROGRAMS DESIGNED TO REDUCE STRESS

Parents of children with developmental disabilities typically report high levels of stress and are at risk for mental health problems such as depressive symptoms. As a consequence, a number of intervention programs have been designed to reduce stress in parents. Following Singer, Ethridge, and Aldana (2007), one may distinguish between three types of stress-reduction programs. Some programs try to reduce psychological distress in parents directly by teaching parents methods for coping with stress. Most of these programs use some form of cognitive–behavioral therapy. Alternatively, some programs are designed to teach parents appropriate skills for interacting effectively with their children, and thus indirectly reduce parent distress. Most of these programs emphasize behavioral skills training. Finally, some programs use a mix of these two approaches.

Singer (2002) made a strong case for intervention studies using randomized experimental designs. Controlled research designs, unlike correlational designs, can rule out, at least provisionally, alternative explanations for outcomes. In addition, key external audiences may not take the results seriously unless the studies use controlled designs. Although we have seen that methodological pluralism (most notably, in the form of narrative studies) has been helpful in the study of disabilities, intervention research should be geared toward determining causal explanations of treatment effects. Accordingly, what follows is a review of studies in which parents were randomly assigned to a treatment or control condition; in many of these studies, control conditions consisted of parents on a waiting list to receive experimental treatments.

Coping Skills Programs

Hastings and Beck (2004) reviewed the literature on intervention programs designed to reduce parenting stress directly. All six studies reviewed found positive results for interventions. For example, Nixon and Singer (1993) randomly assigned mothers of children with disabilities to a cognitive–behavioral group or a waiting list control group. All of the children had severe developmental disabilities; all had intellectual disabilities, and most had other disabling conditions, such as cerebral palsy, autism, epilepsy, or sensory deficits. Intervention included five weekly group sessions aimed at cognitive distortions that contributed to self-blame and guilt. Parents also received homework in the form of monitoring negative thoughts and cognitive distortions and attempting cognitive restructuring. The treatment group showed significant reductions relative to the waiting list group in negative internal attributions, guilt, automatic negative thoughts, and depression.

Greaves (cited in Hastings & Beck, 2004) randomly assigned mothers of children with Down syndrome to rational emotive therapy (RET), applied behavior analysis (ABA), or no treatment control. The first two groups met weekly for 8 weeks. The RET group focused on replacing irrational beliefs with rational beliefs, whereas the ABA group was taught how to apply principles of operant conditioning. Mothers in the RET group reported reduced stress when compared with the other two groups, which did not differ.

Some evidence indicates that stress-reduction treatments produce lasting results. Kirkham (1993) examined the efficacy of a training program in life skills for mothers of children with a variety of developmental disabilities. Mothers were randomly assigned to the skills-building intervention or a parent support group. The skills program included a cognitive–behavioral component designed to reduce stress and depression along with components dedicated to improving communication and problem-solving skills and satisfaction with social support networks. Participants completed measures of stress and depression at pretest, at posttest, and at a 20- to 26-month follow-up. Mothers in the skills-training class reported somewhat lower stress levels at posttest as well as significantly lower depression at follow-up.

Although these studies were successful in reducing parent distress, Hastings and Beck (2004) noted several limitations. First, several of the interventions were broad in nature, making it difficult to isolate the efficacy of cognitive–behavioral treatments, although the Greaves (cited in Hastings & Beck, 2004) study discussed earlier compared RET and ABA. Second, questions about the effectiveness of parental stress interventions for fathers remain. Four of the six studies reported data only for mothers; one study that did report data separately for mothers and fathers showed similar outcomes for the two parents. Third, Hastings and Beck (2004) questioned the clinical significance of the studies. Only one study (Nixon & Singer, 1993) reported effect sizes, and its results suggested small- to medium-size changes on most outcome measures. Finally, the evidence for the long-term effect of these programs is limited due to the small sample sizes in follow-up analyses.

Two recent studies extended these results to families in other countries. Valizadeh, Davaji, and Dadkhah (2009) examined the effectiveness of a coping skills program in Tehran. Mothers of intellectually disabled children were randomly assigned to experimental and control groups. The experimental group received weekly sessions for 12 weeks based on Lazarus and Folkman's (1984) model of cognitive appraisal. Results showed that the stress levels of the experimental but not the control group declined over the 12 weeks. In addition, Wong and Poon (2010) tested the efficacy of a culturally attuned cognitive–behavioral therapy group for Chinese parents of children with developmental disabilities in Melbourne, Australia. Parents were randomly assigned to cognitive–behavioral therapy or waiting list control groups. After 10 weeks of treatment, participants in the therapy group showed significant improvement in measures of general health, parenting stress, and quality of life but not on a measure of dysfunctional attitude.

Parenting Skills Programs

A second set of studies has examined programs that teach parents skills for dealing with behavioral issues in their children. These studies have often used behavioral techniques such as interruption of unwanted behaviors and reinforcement of alternative behaviors. When possible, these programs were integrated into everyday routines such as mealtime, dressing, and bedtime.

These programs have been shown to reduce child misbehavior and thus indirectly parenting stress. Niccols and Mohamed (2000) described an 8-week parent–child interaction skills training group for parents of infants with developmental delay. The program was based on attachment theory. Parents learned skills in reading infant cues via video programs, small group discussions, homework assignments, and peer support. The intervention group showed decreased dysfunctional parent–child interaction, parental distress, sadness/depression, and follow-up service utilization, along with higher levels of consumer satisfaction. For the comparison group, differences between pre- and posttest were not significant.

More recently, McIntyre (2008) used a randomized controlled trial to evaluate a parent training intervention for caregivers of preschool children with developmental disabilities. Families in the experimental group received the usual care plus a 12-week program that included group sessions devoted to play, praise, rewards, the setting of limits, and the handling of challenging behavior. Families in the control group received usual care. Parent intervention was superior to usual care in reducing negative parent–child interactions and child behavior problems. Participants in the experimental group indicated a high degree of satisfaction with the treatment and showed high levels of attendance.

Several studies have found evidence for the maintenance of treatment effects. Pisterman et al. (1989) evaluated a training program for parents of children with attention deficit disorder. Half of the families were randomly assigned to an immediate training program and the other half to a delayed program (i.e., control group). The authors found a positive treatment effect on measures of compliance, parental style of interaction, and management skills. The improvements were maintained at 3-month follow-up. A second study assessed the effect of the program on parent stress on a larger sample of children with attention deficit disorder (Pisterman et al., 1992). Compared with parents awaiting treatment, parents who completed the training reported significant improvement in a measure of parenting stress both immediately after treatment and at 3-month follow up.

Roberts, Mazzucchelli, Studman, and Sanders (2006) examined the efficacy of a 10-session behavioral family intervention for preschoolers with developmental delays. The intervention focused on encouraging the children's development and managing misbehavior. Compared with a waiting list control group, the experimental group was associated with fewer behavioral problems as reported by mothers and independent observers. In addition, both maternal and paternal parenting styles improved, and maternal stress decreased. The gains were maintained at 6-month follow-up. Drew et al. (2002) examined the effectiveness of a parent training intervention for preschool children with autism. In the program, parents were given advice about behavioral management techniques, including reinforcement of appropriate behaviors and interruption of unwanted behaviors. Speech and language consultants visited the home every 6 weeks for 3 hours. The comparison group received therapy services (e.g., speech, occupational) but not parent training. Despite some methodological limitations (e.g., use of parental reports on children's developmental progress), the results indicated that children in the parent training group made more progress than did children in the comparison group at a 12-month follow-up.

Quinn, Carr, Carroll, and O'Sullivan (2007) reported similar results. They compared pre- and posttreatment assessments for parents of preschool children with developmental disabilities and significant behavioral problems. The treatment group was compared with a control group of families on a waiting list. The treatment consisted of a group-based parent training package that involved video modeling. The treatment group showed better adjustment on posttreatment measures than did the control group, and gains were maintained at a 10-month follow-up.

The strongest evidence for the long-term effects of parent training programs comes from Feldman and Werner (2002), who evaluated collateral effects of behavioral parent training on families with children who had developmental disabilities and behavior disorders. The intervention consisted of 1- to 2-hour weekly home visits by a behavioral consultant that generally lasted 3 to 6 months. They compared 18 behavioral parent training graduates with 18 similar families waiting for service. Training graduates reported significantly less child behavior problems, disruptions to child and family quality of life, and stress related to limits on family opportunities. These results were maintained up to 5 years after discharge. Graduates also reported higher levels of self-efficacy in stopping child behavior problems, preventing new occurrences, and teaching children appropriate behaviors.

Mixed Programs

Several programs included a mix of stress reduction and parenting techniques. Salt et al. (2002) evaluated the effectiveness of a developmentally based early intervention program for autism. The program was modeled on the Scottish Centre for Autism treatment program. Parents were trained to interpret child behavior as potential interaction and to shape the child's interactions. In addition, parent support groups were offered. Results indicated that children in the treatment group improved significantly more than those in the control group on measures of joint attention, social interaction, imitation, daily living skills, motor skills, and an adaptive behavior composite. Parents in the treatment group, but not those in the control group, showed a reduction in total stress. Hudson et al. (2003) evaluated an intervention program for parents of children with intellectual disability and challenging behaviors. The program was based on an approach that emphasized child behavior management as well as stress management. Following the program, parents reported that they were less stressed, felt more efficacious about managing their child's behavior, and were less hassled about meeting their own needs; in addition, they reported that their children's behavior had improved. Families generally reported high levels of satisfaction with the content and delivery of the materials.

Bristol, Gallagher, and Holt (1993) included several components in a program to address depressive symptoms of mothers of young children with autism. Mothers were trained to carry out and evaluate behavior modification techniques through one-on-one modeling, reinforcement, and guided feedback. In addition, components addressed home environment management and parent attitude adaptation. Mothers in the treatment group declined in depressive symptoms relative to a comparison group, and the gains were maintained in a follow-up 18 months later.

There is further indication that such gains are enduring. Tonge et al. (2006) combined parent education and behavior management in an intervention program for parents of preschool children with autism. A comparison group received counseling and parent education. Both treatments resulted in significant and progressive improvement in overall mental health at follow up. The parent education and behavior management intervention was effective in alleviating a greater percentage of anxiety, insomnia, and somatic symptoms and family dysfunction than parent education and counseling at a 6-month follow-up.

Meta-Analyses

One of the concerns noted by Hastings and Beck (2004) was the clinical significance of the results in these treatment studies. A pair of meta-analyses examined the effect sizes of various studies. Barlow, Coren, and Stewart-Brown (2002) conducted a meta-analysis of the effectiveness of parenting programs in the United Kingdom in improving maternal psychosocial health. A total of 23 studies met the inclusion criteria, and 17 provided sufficient data on the five outcomes of interest: depression, anxiety, self-esteem, social support, and relationship with partner. Results were significant for depression, anxiety, self-esteem, and relationship with partner. The results for social support were not significant. Follow-up data were also encouraging. The authors concluded that parenting programs make a significant contribution to the short-term psychosocial health of mothers. One limitation of the Barlow et al. article, for our purposes, is that only some of the studies in the meta-analysis were directly relevant to families of children with developmental disorders; other studies pertained to children with conduct disorders or "perceived problems."

Singer, Ethridge, and Aldana (2007) conducted a meta-analysis of group intervention research for parents of children with developmental disorders. The 17 studies were grouped into three categories: parenting education studies involving behavioral parent training, coping skills education studies based primarily on cognitive–behavioral training, and mixed studies. Consistent reductions in parental distress were associated with all three types of programs. Singer et al. (2007) reported that the overall effect size for all 17 studies was $d = 0.29$. The effect size was larger for the multicomponent programs (0.90) than for programs that were exclusively ABA (0.25) or cognitive–behavioral therapy (0.34). Singer et al. (2007) also noted some limitations in their review. Most of the parents in these studies were White and middle class. In addition, most of the studies were short term, and the samples were limited in size. Nonetheless, Singer et al. (2007) suggest that the studies meet the criteria for evidence-based practice, at least for middle-class mothers in the short term. The effect of interventions for fathers, while more limited, was also encouraging.

On balance, these studies indicate that programs designed to reduce parenting stress can be effective. Both coping skills and parent training programs have been shown to be effective in reducing parenting stress, and there is evidence that a combination of the two types of programs is the most effective treatment. Moreover, the studies indicate that the gains that parents receive in these programs are enduring.

INTERVENTION PROGRAMS DESIGNED TO INCREASE POSITIVE EMOTIONS

Is it possible not only to reduce stress but also to promote happiness and life satisfaction? We now turn to interventions based on positive psychology. Although there are few data, there are reasons to think that positive psychology interventions may be effective for families of children with developmental disabilities. First, a number of studies show successful positive psychology interventions, particularly for individuals with depressive symptoms. Since parents of children with disabilities are at risk for depression, it seems reasonable to expect that these treatments would be effective for this population. Second, the few studies that have applied positive psychology principles to families of children with disabilities have reported promising results.

Positive Psychology Interventions

Studies of the effectiveness of intervention programs based on positive psychology principles have become popular in recent years. Reviews of the rapidly developing literature have been published (Duckworth, Steen, & Seligman, 2005; Layous, Chancellor, Lyubomirsky, Wang, & Doraiswamy, 2011; Sin & Lyubomirsky, 2009). The effectiveness of positive psychology interventions in reducing depression, increasing psychological well-being, or both has been explored.

Consider first the evidence regarding depression. Mindfulness interventions may be effective in reducing depression (Grossman, Tiefenthaler-Gilmer, Raysz, & Kesper, 2007; Zautra et al., 2008). Grossman et al. (2007) examined the effectiveness of a mindfulness-based stress reduction program on clients with fibromyalgia. The intervention included a variety of mindfulness practices, including yoga and the use of mindfulness in stressful social situations. Relative to a social support condition, participants in the mindfulness group showed greater reductions in pain, anxiety, and depression, and the reductions were sustained in a 3-year follow-up analysis. Similarly, Zautra et al. (2008) found some evidence of the effectiveness of mindfulness interventions in reducing pain and depression in clients with rheumatoid arthritis. Individuals receiving mindfulness treatments showed greater reduction in pain than did a group receiving education, although less reduction in pain than did a cognitive–behavioral treatment group. With regard to depression, the mindfulness treatment was most effective. Moreover, patients with a history of depression benefited the most from the mindfulness treatment. Thus, the relative value of mindfulness and cognitive behavioral treatments depended on the outcome measure.

Forgiveness treatments for reducing depression have also been shown to be effective. S. R. Freedman and Enright (1996) randomly assigned incest survivors to a weekly forgiveness intervention or a waiting list control group. The intervention encouraged individuals to recognize their emotional responses and to express empathy and compassion for the offenders. Following the intervention, the experimental group achieved gains in forgiveness and hope and saw reductions in depression and anxiety relative to the control group. Reed and Enright (2006) found similar results with spousal abuse victims.

With regard to well-being, in some of the earliest studies of happiness intervention, Fordyce (1977, 1983) randomly assigned community college classes to an intervention with detailed strategies for increasing happiness (e.g., keep busy, be more active, spend more time socializing) and several control groups. Students in the intervention group were happier, less anxious, and less depressed at the end of the term. Most participants who completed the survey 9 to 18 months later reported continued happiness increases. Although limited, this research suggests that happiness can be increased.

Emmons and McCullough (2003) explored the effectiveness of gratitude interventions for increasing happiness and well-being. Undergraduate students and individuals with neuromuscular disease were randomly assigned to one of several conditions. Those in the gratitude condition were asked to identify five things that they were grateful or thankful for over the past week (i.e., "count your blessings"). Other participants either identified current hassles or current events without specifying whether they were positive or negative. Individuals then recorded their moods, physical symptoms, and overall life satisfaction. The gratitude condition displayed heightened well-being on most but not all measures. Similarly, Lyubomirsky, Sheldon, and Schkade (2005) found that participants who counted their blessings or performed acts of kindness improved their well-being over a 6-week intervention period. The timing of these acts mattered. When individuals distributed these acts over a week, there was little change, but when they engaged in the same number of acts all in the same day, there was improvement in well-being. Lyubomirsky and colleagues speculated that since many of the kind acts that individuals performed were minor, spreading them out over a period of a week might have diminished their impact.

Several studies have found that writing about positive events can lead to a short-term boost in mood (Burton & King, 2004, 2008; Pennebaker & Francis, 1996). Burton and King (2004) randomly assigned undergraduates to write about either an intensely positive experience or a control topic for 20 minutes each day for 3 consecutive days. Writing about intensely positive experiences lifted mood and was associated with fewer health center visits 3 months later. A subsequent study (Burton & King, 2008) found that even a very brief writing exercise was productive. Participants wrote about either a personal trauma, a positive life experience, or a control topic for 2 minutes per day for 2 days. Both the trauma and the positive experience writing led to fewer reported health complaints 4 to 6 weeks later.

Seligman, Steen, Park, and Peterson (2005) compared the effectiveness of five positive psychology interventions with a placebo control exercise for both increasing happiness and reducing depression by using an Internet study. Individuals completed measures of happiness and depression online. Of the five exercises, two—*using signature strengths in a new way* and *identifying three good things in life*—produced lasting change 6 months after the intervention. The *using signature strengths in a new way* exercise asked participants to complete a questionnaire that identified their strengths and then asked respondents to use one of their strengths in a new and different way every day for a week. The *identifying three good things in life* exercise asked participants to write down three things that went well each day and their causes every night for 1 week. Participants in these two conditions were happier and less depressed. Two other exercises and the placebo control created positive but transient effects on happiness and depressive symptoms. In addition, the participants who continued the intervention beyond 1 week (the amount of time requested) had continued increased happiness and decreased depressive symptoms at the 1-month follow-up.

Seligman, Rashid, and Parks (2006) conducted an Internet study with self-selected depressed individuals. Positive psychotherapy consisted of a series of exercises, including using your strengths, gratitude visits (writing a letter of gratitude to a person one has not properly thanked), and savoring (taking the time, once a day, to enjoy something one usually hurries through, such as a shower). Positive psychotherapy delivered to groups reduced depressive symptoms at 1-year follow-up. Satisfaction with life was also somewhat improved for the positive intervention group. A second study examined positive psychotherapy delivered to individuals. Relative to treatment as usual, with or without medication, the positive psychotherapy led to more reduction in depression and enhanced happiness.

Sin and Lyubomirsky (2009) conducted a meta-analysis of positive psychology interventions. The meta-analysis included 51 interventions with a total of 4,266 individuals. Results revealed that positive psychology interventions significantly enhanced well-being and decreased depressive symptoms. Of 49 studies on well-being, 96% of the effect sizes were in the predicted direction. In addition, 80% of the 25 studies on depression favored positive psychology interventions. A number of variables influenced the effectiveness of the interventions, including depression status, self-selection, and age of the participants along with the format and duration of the interventions. Depressed individuals benefited more from these interventions than nondepressed individuals, and self-selected participants gained more than non-self-selected counterparts. A trend for more successful interventions in older participants was found. Individual therapy was also more effective than group-administered treatment. The authors encouraged clinicians to incorporate positive psychology interventions, particularly those geared at individuals rather than groups and for a longer period of time, into their clinical practice.

Although positive psychology interventions have been shown to be generally effective, there are exceptions. We previously considered the potential downside in optimism as a form of maladaptive persistence (see Chapter 3, this volume). Similar observations apply to other positive psychology constructs such as kindness and forgiveness. For example, McNulty (2010) found that the effect of positive interventions for married couples depended on the level of marital problems. Positive interventions were most effective for couples that experienced infrequent or minor problems. Positive interventions were less effective for couples facing major problems; these couples benefited more from approaches that addressed the negative aspects of their relationships. These results remind us that the efficacy of positive psychology interventions, like any treatment, must be viewed in context.

Implications for Parents of Children With Disabilities

Few attempts have been made to apply positive psychology interventions to parents of children with developmental disabilities, but the early results are promising. Cosden, Koegel, Koegel, Greenwell, and Klein (2006) endorsed strength-based assessment for children with autism spectrum disorders. These assessments emphasized what a child can do as opposed to what the child cannot do. Cosden et al. did not argue that strength-based approaches should supplant more traditional approaches; rather, they suggested that strength-based assessments could provide a useful complement to more traditional deficit-based assessment approaches by helping mental health professionals identify and utilize strengths in developing intervention strategies for children with disabilities.

Strength-based approaches may be a good fit with approaches that emphasize partnerships between professionals and parents. Steiner, Koegel, Koegel, and Ence (2012) discussed the application of strength-based approaches to the education of parents of children with autism. Although parent education is a ubiquitous component of comprehensive programs for children with autism spectrum disorder, the most effective form of parent education is less clear. Steiner et al. (2012) suggested that such education should emphasize behavioral goal setting and involve parents in decision making, including what to work on during weekly sessions and how to go about it. This type of approach may be particularly appropriate for parents of children with autism, given the uncertainty and stress associated with autism spectrum disorder.

Four studies to date have specifically examined the effectiveness of a strength-based approach to parent education for children with autism. Steiner (2011) used an alternating treatment design to compare the effects of therapist statements that dealt with the child's deficits against therapist statements that emphasized strengths. For example, a deficit statement might be that it is difficult to gain the child's attention and he does not focus on any one thing for very long, whereas a strength statement would be that the child has a lot of interests, which is a good sign. The results indicated that when parents received the strength-based approach they made more positive statements about their child and exhibited more physical affection toward their child.

More recently, Benn, Akiva, Arel, and Roeser (2012) examined the effects of mindfulness training for parents of children with special educational needs. They randomly assigned parents to treatment and control conditions. For the mindfulness treatment, parents attended training sessions twice a week for 5 weeks. The training included sessions on exploring forgiveness, working with conflict and anger, and developing compassion and kindness. Parents completed measures of well-being and caregiving competence prior to the program, at program completion, and in a follow-up 2 months later. Mindfulness training had a statistically significant effect on 7 of 8 measures of psychological well-being, with six findings significant at follow-up. However, measures of parenting self-efficacy and the quality of parent–child interaction did not show significant effects. The results suggest that mindfulness training has a positive benefit on stress reduction in parents. However, further research will be needed to determine to what extent the reduction in stress influences parent–child interaction.

There is clearly a need for additional research in this area. Several approaches may be considered. First, the efficacy of positive psychology interventions for reducing depression symptoms in parents of children with disabilities should be investigated. Studies reviewed in Chapter 3 indicate that parents of children with developmental disabilities experience high levels of stress and are at risk for stress-related depressive symptoms. Positive psychology interventions may be beneficial in reducing these parenting-based depressive symptoms.

Second, the efficacy of happiness interventions for parents of children with disabilities should be explored. Studies of parent narratives reviewed in Chapters 9 and 10 indicated that some parents, despite significant levels of stress, achieve positive outcomes on their own. Nonetheless, happiness and mindfulness interventions may be useful in assisting other parents in identifying benefits associated with parenting a child with a developmental disability. In addition, further analysis of successful self-adopted happiness strategies should inform future efforts to develop positive psychology interventions.

Third, some of the specific positive psychology interventions, such as using signature strengths in a new way, may be particularly appropriate for these parents. For example, parents of children with disabilities may develop character strengths such as courage and wisdom but may be uncertain how to share or employ them. Professional guidance to assist parents in translating these strengths into new contexts might be appropriate.

12

CONCLUSIONS AND FUTURE DIRECTIONS

In this chapter, I identify and briefly discuss some conclusions that appear to be well established by research covered in this volume. I then identify some questions that are not fully resolved by present research but that could become fruitful lines of inquiry.

CONCLUSIONS

The immediate experience of discovering that one's child has a developmental disability comes as a shock to many parents, and their subsequent emotional experience is similar to posttraumatic stress disorder.

As discussed in Chapter 2, the parents of infants in a newborn intensive care unit are initially overwhelmed by the gravity of their infant's condition and the hospital environment. Retrospective studies indicate that the parents may experience symptoms similar to posttraumatic stress disorder.

http://dx.doi.org/10.1037/14192-012
Families of Children With Developmental Disabilities: Understanding Stress and Opportunities for Growth,
by D. W. Carroll

Parents may relive the traumatic event and maintain high levels of emotional arousal. In addition, the stress experienced by the parents influences early parent–child interactions and may contribute to sleeping and eating issues in infants. Studies have found that parents continue to experience elevated levels of stress 2 to 3 years following their hospital experience.

Parents of children with developmental disabilities experience significant and enduring levels of stress and are at risk for depressive symptoms.

The ongoing stress of caring for a child with a disability influences parents emotionally, socially, and financially. Research in Chapter 3 indicates that parents with severe and enduring levels of stress are at risk for depressive symptoms, although not necessarily clinical depression. Estimates are that 25% to 30% of parents of children with developmental disabilities will experience heightened levels of depressive symptoms. Preexisting familial characteristics may play a role as well; parents of children with autism spectrum disorder (ASD) who have subclinical levels of autistic symptoms are more at risk for developing depressive symptoms.

Parents of children with disabilities typically show high levels of optimism, and those parents who display optimism fare better than those who do not.

Studies reviewed in Chapter 3 indicate that parents of children with developmental disabilities often possess high levels of optimism. Research also reveals that optimism may moderate the relationship between stress and both physical and psychological health by serving as a buffer against stress. Moreover, optimism may mediate the relationship between social support and maternal well-being. There is continued discussion regarding the boundary between adaptive forms of optimism and maladaptive persistence.

Narratives of parents of children with disabilities reveal positive outcomes, including a desire for constructing meaning from difficult life experiences.

As seen in Chapter 9, parents often construct meaningful stories from their experiences that intermix sorrow, anger, and joy. Parent narratives emphasize the stresses of being a caregiver and tensions with professionals along with a sense of optimism, a desire to give back to others, and an interest in constructing meaning from their experiences. Happiness and life satisfaction are related to the ability of parents to divest prior expectations and invest resources into new dreams for their children and themselves.

Children with disabilities influence the entire family by altering family routines and roles, which leads to new challenges for parents, siblings, and grandparents.

Families thrive on the roles and routines that maintain the family system, but it is more difficult for families of children with developmental disabilities to establish these types of regularity. Parents often feel a strain in establishing balance between family and work responsibilities and in identifying different roles within the family. Mothers typically carry the heaviest burden in caring for children with disabilities. Young siblings may feel resentment regarding the parental attention devoted to their siblings with disabilities or the care-giving and household responsibilities they are expected to assume. As a consequence, some siblings experience adjustment problems. Grandparents may feel unprepared for their new role and may not be able to provide sufficient emotional support to their adult children.

For parents of children with developmental disabilities, the challenge of securing medical services and equipment is a major source of stress.

Many of the concerns with medical professionals arise from difficulties in coordinating medical care and the need for more family-centered care. Coordination of care is a significant hassle for many families, as parents may need to arrange multiple appointments with several health care providers. Many families experience financial distress as a consequence of their child's disability and have unmet health care needs. In addition, parents face the challenge of learning how to communicate with physicians to secure medical services and equipment for their children.

Parents of children with developmental disabilities are often dissatisfied with educational professionals who serve their children.

Parents have considerable trust issues with teachers and other educational professionals who, they believe, often hold attitudes that are not conducive to their child's development. In particular, parents frequently prefer a more inclusive form of education for their children than educational professionals are prepared to provide. In addition, parents of children with autism are increasingly unhappy with the level and quality of services available for their children. As a consequence of these interactions, some parents become advocates for educational change within the school system and beyond.

Families who care for children with developmental disabilities often suffer social exclusion, due to both ignorance and stigma.

For many parents of children with disabilities, the response of society at large is at least as troubling as their children's medical or behavioral issues. Individuals with disabilities are often marginalized in society, and those who are associated with them also experience stigmatization and social exclusion. Social exclusion leads to impairments in self-regulation and difficulty in performing complex cognitive tasks. As a consequence of their social exclusion, parents often turn to other parents of children with disabilities, who may be able to provide forms of social support that family members and friends cannot provide.

Parents who have strong social support systems fare better than those who do not.

Parents who have reliable instrumental and emotional support from family members, friends, and other parents of children with disabilities have fewer adverse consequences than those who do not. Social support moderates the link between stress and depressive symptoms. Both quantitative and qualitative research suggest that parent support programs (particularly programs that match parents whose children have similar conditions) can be an important adjunct to traditional professional services.

New challenges arise for both parents and individuals with disabilities as these individuals grow into their later adolescent and early adult years.

As they enter adolescence and early adulthood, youths with disabilities encounter new questions regarding future employment, continued education, and independent living. Their parents provide support and assistance in all of these endeavors. When youths with disabilities leave the home, the level of daily stress for parents may be lessened, but typically there is still considerable contact between family members. The long-term impact of part-time employment causes financial strain for parents, particularly mothers, at midlife. Parents of individuals with disabilities often experience poorer mental health at midlife than does the general population. The psychological well-being of parents is related to their relationship with their adult children as well as to the children's success in attaining societal measures of adult status.

As individuals with disabilities move into adulthood, some of their siblings willingly take on significant responsibilities in caring for them as well as advocacy roles.

Compared with siblings of young adults with mental illness, siblings of young adults with intellectual disabilities remain in closer contact with their sisters and brothers, both emotionally and geographically. Siblings of young adults with disabilities value their relationships with their brothers and sisters. Some siblings choose over time to become advocates for their sisters and brothers, including advocating for change in various social systems. There is, however, considerable variability in the degree to which siblings take on daily caregiving responsibilities in regard to their brothers or sisters and how siblings balance their relationships with their brothers and sisters with their own family life.

When a child with disabilities dies, parents often experience patterns of grief that are difficult for other people to understand and appreciate fully.

Despite their children's health issues, parents of children with developmental disabilities are often surprised by their child's death, which they frequently experience as sudden or unexpected. Many parents experience a double transition: accepting that their child has a disability and then transitioning to a life without that child. Parents' challenges in adapting to their loss are complicated by the fact that many friends and family members have difficulty appreciating the loss, thus contributing to an ongoing sense of social isolation.

Intervention programs that include stress reduction techniques and parenting skills training have been found to reduce child behavioral issues and parenting stress.

Meta-analyses reviewed in Chapter 11 indicate that programs designed to reduce parenting stress are effective. Programs that teach cognitive–behavioral techniques reduce stress in parents, and those that teach applied behavioral analysis techniques reduce child behavioral issues as well as parenting stress. Effect sizes indicate that a combination of the two techniques is more effective than either in isolation.

FUTURE DIRECTIONS

Intervention programs for parents of infants in newborn intensive care units should be expanded to examine longer term outcomes.

Current intervention programs for parents of infants in newborn intensive care units are limited to educating parents about infant behavior and assessing short-term parental outcomes. Development and evaluation of programs aimed at assessing longer-term parental functioning and addressing posttraumatic symptoms in parents of children in newborn intensive care units are needed.

Studies of parental responses to diagnoses of Down syndrome and ASD need to be extended to diagnoses of other disabilities.

From a diagnostic perspective, Down syndrome and ASD present a stark contrast. Parents learn of the diagnosis of Down syndrome very early in their child's life, whereas parents of children with ASD typically do not receive this diagnosis until the child is 5 or 6 years old, and often only after multiple medical appointments. Parental resolution of a child's diagnosis with a disability appears to be related to diagnostic uncertainty, with parents of children with ASD exhibiting lower levels of resolution. These disabilities probably occupy two ends of a continuum pertaining to the degree of uncertainty associated with a child's diagnosis. Further exploration of the entire continuum would be fruitful.

There is a need to more comprehensively research the similarities as well as differences in family responses to various developmental disabilities.

Research on how different disabilities influence the family is fragmentary and unconnected. Although considerable research has examined the behavioral issues associated with ASD and spina bifida, less is known about how other aspects of family experience may be influenced by the nature of the child's disability. For example, little research has looked at the influence of optimism or compared sibling relationships as a function of disability type. Further research that clarifies both similarities and differences between the family experiences with various disabilities is needed to develop a comprehensive account of how child disability influences family functioning.

Although it is clear that some parents may experience positive benefit from the stress of caring for a child with disabilities, a fuller understanding of when and how these benefits may be derived is in order.

Studies discussed in Chapter 3 have found that parents of children with disabilities may find meaning and benefit in their parenting experience. Such studies provide a useful antidote to the prevalent conclusion that these parents suffer from unrelenting stress. However, we do not currently know how frequently meaning- and benefit-finding responses occur or what personality, family, or environmental factors might influence them. Moreover, although there has been some recent effort to link these studies with the theoretical framework of positive psychology, more integration along this line would be helpful.

There is a need for additional research on the reactions of grandparents to their new roles, and in particular on the relationship between grandparents and grandchildren with disabilities.

Grandparents may play multiple roles in the families of children with disabilities. They may provide emotional and instrumental support for parents as well as establishing relationships with their grandchildren. However, grandparents, no less than parents, need to adjust to unexpected life circumstances and may need help in redefining their role within the family. These issues are deserving of additional scrutiny.

The study of medical communication between parent, child, and physician holds much promise, but at present the research is fragmentary and does not fully identify the impact of communication issues.

Research reviewed in Chapter 5 indicates that medical communication issues may play an important role in parents' ability to secure appropriate medical services and equipment for their children. However, most of the research on medical discourse analysis deals with parents of children without disabilities. The impact of communication issues has not been sufficiently explored within the disability field.

There are significant gaps in our knowledge about how parents work with educational professionals, how they resolve their differences, and how these discussions influence the child's educational progress.

The research discussed in Chapter 6 indicates that trust issues plague the relationships between parents and educational professionals. Parents generally prefer an inclusive approach to educating children with disabilities, an approach that many professionals regard as dubious, particularly when it is applied to children with severe disabilities. Studies of different attitudes regarding inclusive education and the conflicts that they create should be complemented with research that examines how (and how well) parents and educational professionals work together in the planning for the education of children with disabilities.

Research on family quality of life shows considerable promise for understanding the global aspects of family functioning for families touched by disability.

Increasing interest in the global concept of family quality of life has led to the creation of several instruments designed to assess family functioning in multiple domains such as family interaction, emotional well-being, and social support. These instruments provide a more comprehensive view of family processes than do many of the measures commonly used in research on families with disabilities. Use of such instruments has the potential to contribute to a more well-rounded view of family functioning than is currently available.

Presently, narrative studies of parents are primarily descriptive, and there is a need to pursue relationships between narrative themes and psychological measures of well-being, life satisfaction, and happiness.

The majority of narrative studies have been concerned with identifying themes that are pervasive in the stories that parents tell. Although these narratives are vivid, there is a need to determine how parental stories influence personal and family functioning. A mixture of qualitative and quantitative methods can be especially useful in determining the psychological impact of different narrative strategies. In particular, additional research on how different narrative themes might predict life satisfaction and happiness is warranted.

There is a need for additional research on bereavement in parents of children with disabilities and to connect the research better with contemporary psychological models of bereavement.

As noted in Chapter 10, contemporary theories of bereavement have emphasized the diversity of bereavement responses and, in particular, the frequency of resilience in bereaved spouses. Research on bereavement in parents of children with disabilities has not been closely tied to the broader bereavement literature. In particular, studies of bereavement in parents have not included longitudinal studies that permit inferences regarding the salience of various psychological responses over time. In addition, comparisons of parents of children with disabilities with groups such as caregivers of elderly family members and parents of typically developing children who have died in accidents would be helpful in determining the causal connections between different aspects of the parenting experience and corresponding bereavement responses.

Graduate programs in clinical psychology do not provide sufficient training in disabilities.

There is a clear need for additional coursework in graduate programs in clinical psychology on disability issues in general and on family responses to childhood disability in particular. Despite federal legislation that has drawn attention to disability issues, graduate coursework in disability issues is insufficient and too often focused on the medical model to the exclusion of the social aspects of disability.

Research on the efficacy of programs designed to reduce parenting stress need to include more fathers and more longer-term assessments.

The research that has evaluated the effectiveness of stress reduction programs, along with most of the research discussed in this book, has focused primarily on mothers. Mothers bear a disproportionate burden in the care of children with disabilities and provide the most convenient samples for researchers. Nonetheless, fathers' experiences and emotional responses may differ from those of mothers, and treatment programs that are most efficacious for fathers may differ from those designed for mothers. In addition, much of the research on program efficacy has used short-term assessments. Although it is encouraging to see positive results in follow-up assessments 6 months or a year later, longer-term follow-up assessments would be beneficial.

Studies of positive psychotherapy for depression are promising, but there is a need for research on these interventions directly with parents of children with developmental disabilities.

Positive psychotherapy has been found to be effective in reducing depressive symptoms. Since parents of children with disabilities are at risk for depressive symptoms, there is reason to think that positive psychology interventions would be beneficial for this population. In addition, positive psychology interventions, including those related to finding personal strengths, have been found to promote both happiness and life satisfaction. There is a need to apply the positive psychology framework to the study of families of children with disabilities. The research to date is promising but limited.

It is clear from the review of research in the preceding chapters that a great deal of knowledge has been accumulated about the experiences of families of children with developmental disabilities. The emergence of a research-based consensus on a number of issues is extremely encouraging. At the same time, the success of many research programs has opened areas for future work. To a significant extent, these initiatives focus on the degree to which the findings to date generalize equally well to individuals with different disabilities and to families from different racial and ethnic backgrounds. These emerging lines of study should enrich our understanding of the multiple ways that children with disabilities influence family functioning.

Although there is always a need for more studies, existing research is sufficient to provide evidence-based recommendations on a number of issues that can contribute to the quality of life for families of children with disabilities. They include, but are not limited to, the value of peer support groups for parents, the efficacy of stress reduction programs, and the special challenges associated with losing a child with a developmental disability. I hope that the research consensus outlined in the preceding pages will be useful in helping to develop support programs that both maintain and improve the quality of life for families of individuals with disabilities.

REFERENCES

Abbeduto, L., Seltzer, M. M., Shattuck, P., Krauss, M. W., Orsmond, G., & Murphy, M. M. (2004). Psychological well-being and coping in mothers of youth with autism, Down syndrome, or fragile X syndrome. *American Journal on Mental Retardation, 109,* 237–254. Retrieved from http://www.waisman.wisc.edu/family/pubs/autism/2004%20Abbeduto%20Seltzer%20Shattuck%20psyc%20well%20being.pdf

Abelson, A. G. (1999). Respite care needs of parents of children with developmental disabilities. *Focus on Autism and Other Developmental Disabilities, 14,* 96–100. doi:10.1177/108835769901400204

Abrams, E. Z., & Goodman, J. F. (1998). Diagnosing developmental problems in children: Parents and professionals negotiate bad news. *Journal of Pediatric Psychology, 23,* 87–98. doi:10.1093/jpepsy/23.2.87

Adams, S. H., Newacheck, P. W., Park, J., Brindis, C. D., & Irwin, C. E. (2007). Health insurance across vulnerable ages: Patterns and disparities from adolescence to the early 30s. *Pediatrics, 119,* e1033–e1039. doi:10.1542/peds.2006-1730

Agran, M., Alper, S., & Wehmeyer, M. (2002). Access to the general curriculum for students with significant disabilities: What it means to teachers. *Education & Training in Mental Retardation & Developmental Disabilities, 37,* 123–133. Retrieved from http://www.nytransition.org/resources/search

Åhlund, S., Clarke, P., Hill, J., & Thalange, N. K. S. (2009). Post-traumatic stress symptoms in mothers of very low birth weight infant 2–3 years post-partum. *Archives of Women's Mental Health, 12,* 261–264. doi:10.1007/s00737-009-0067-4

Ainbinder, J. G., Blanchard, L. W., Singer, G. H. S., Sullivan, M. E., Powers, L. K., Marquis, J. G., . . . Santelli, B. (1998). A qualitative study of parent to parent support for parents of children with special needs. *Journal of Pediatric Psychology, 23,* 99–109. doi:10.1093/jpepsy/23.2.99

Akrami, N., Ekehammar, B., & Bergh, R. (2011). Generalized prejudice: Common and specific components. *Psychological Science, 22,* 57–59. doi:10.1177/0956797610390384

American Academy of Pediatrics. (2002). The medical home. *Pediatrics, 110*(1), 184–186. doi:10.1542/peds.110.1.184

American Psychiatric Association. (2000). *Diagnostic and statistical manual of mental disorders* (4th ed., text rev.). Washington, DC: Author.

American Psychological Association. (2012). Guidelines for assessment of and intervention with persons with disabilities. *American Psychologist, 67,* 43–62. doi:10.1037/a0025892

Americans With Disabilities Act of 1990, as amended, 42 U. S. C. A. 12101 et seq. Retrieved from http://www.ada.gov/pubs/ada.htm

Anastopolous, A. D., Guevremont, D. C., Shelton, T. L., & DuPaul, G. J. (1992). Parenting stress among families of children with attention deficit hyperactivity disorder. *Journal of Abnormal Child Psychology, 20,* 503–520. doi:10.1007/BF00916812

Armstrong, M. I., Birnie-Lefcovitch, S., & Ungar, M. T. (2005). Pathways between social support, family well being, quality of parenting, and child resilience: What we know. *Journal of Child and Family Studies, 14,* 269–281. doi:10.1007/s10826-005-5054-4

Attig, T. (2004). Disenfranchised grief revisited: Discounting hope and love. *Omega—Journal of Death and Dying, 49,* 197–215. doi:10.2190/P4TT-J3BF-KFDR-5JB1

Bachner, Y. G., Carmel, S., Lubetzky, H., Heiman, N., & Galil, A. (2006). Parent–therapist communication and satisfaction with the services of a child development center: A comparison between Israeli parents—Jews and Bedouins. *Health Communication, 19,* 221–229. doi:10.1207/s15327027hc1903_4

Baergen, R. (2006). How hopeful is too hopeful? Responding to unreasonably optimistic parents. *Pediatric Nursing, 32,* 482–486. Retrieved from http://www.sonoma.edu/users/c/catlin/edited_articles/Edited%20Baergen%20Hope.pdf

Bailey, D. B., Jr., Golden, R. N., Roberts, J., & Ford, A. (2007). Maternal depression and developmental disability: Research critique. *Mental Retardation and Developmental Disabilities Research Reviews, 13,* 321–329. doi:10.1002/mrdd.20172

Bailey, D. B., Skinner, D., & Sparkman, K. L. (2003). Discovering fragile X syndrome: Family experiences and perceptions. *Pediatrics, 111,* 407–416. doi:10.1542/peds.111.2.407

Baker, B. L., Blacher, J., & Olsson, M. B. (2005). Preschool children with and without developmental delay: Behavioural problems, parents' optimism and well-being. *Journal of Intellectual Disability Research, 49,* 575–590. doi:10.1111/j.1365-2788.2005.00691.x

Baker, B. L., McIntyre, L. L., Blacher, J., Crnic, K., Edelbrock, C., & Low, C. (2003). Pre-school children with and without developmental delay: Behaviour problems and parenting stress over time. *Journal of Intellectual Disability Research, 47,* 217–230. doi:10.1046/j.1365-2788.2003.00484.x

Baker, D. L., Miller, E., Dang, M. T., Yaangh, C.-S., & Hansen, R. L. (2010). Developing culturally responsive approaches with Southeast Asian American families experiencing developmental disabilities. *Pediatrics, 126,* S146–S150. doi:10.1542/peds.2010-1466I

Baker, J. K., Smith, L. E., Greenberg, J. S., Seltzer, M. M., & Taylor, J. L. (2011). Change in maternal criticism and behavior problems in adolescents and adults with autism across a 7-year period. *Journal of Abnormal Psychology, 120,* 465–475. doi:10.1037/a0021900

Barak-Levy, Y., Goldstein, E., & Weinstock, M. (2010). Adjustment characteristics of healthy siblings of children with autism. *Journal of Family Studies, 16,* 155–164. doi:10.5172/jfs.16.2.155

Barlow, J., Coren, E., & Stewart-Brown, S. (2002). Meta-analysis of the effectiveness of parenting programmes in improving maternal psychosocial health. *The British Journal of General Practice, 52*, 223–233. Retrieved from http://www.ncbi.nlm. nih.gov/pmc/issues/125152/

Barnett, D., Clements, M., Kaplan-Estrin, M., & Fialka, J. (2003). Building new dreams: Supporting parents' adaptation to their child with special needs. *Infants and Young Children, 16*, 184–200. doi:10.1097/00001163-200307000-00002

Bauer, J. J., & Bonanno, G. A. (2001). Continuity amid discontinuity: Bridging one's past and present in stories of conjugal bereavement. *Narrative Inquiry, 11*, 123–158. doi:10.1075/ni.11.1.06bau

Bauer, J. J., & McAdams, D. P. (2004). Personal growth in adults' stories of life transitions. *Journal of Personality, 72*, 573–602. doi:10.1111/j.0022-3506.2004.00273.x

Baumeister, R. F., DeWall, C. N., Ciarocco, N. J., & Twenge, J. M. (2005). Social exclusion impairs self-regulation. *Journal of Personality and Social Psychology, 88*, 589–604. doi:10.1037/0022-3514.88.4.589

Baumeister, R. F., Twenge, J. M., & Nuss, C. K. (2002). Effects of social exclusion on cognitive processes: Anticipated aloneness reduces intelligent thought. *Journal of Personality and Social Psychology, 83*, 817–827. doi:10.1037/ 0022-3514.83.4.817

Baumrind, D. (1971). Current patterns of parental authority. *Developmental Psychology, 4*, 1–103. doi:10.1037/h0030372

Bellin, M. H., & Rice, K. M. (2009). Individual, family, and peer factors associated with the quality of sibling relationships in families of youths with spina bifida. *Journal of Family Psychology, 23*, 39–47. doi:10.1037/a0014381

Belsky, J., & Pluess, M. (2009). Beyond diathesis stress: Differential susceptibility to environmental influences. *Psychological Bulletin, 135*, 885–908. doi:10.1037/ a0017376

Benn, R., Akiva, T., Arel, S., & Roeser, R. W. (2012). Mindfulness training effects for parents and educators of children with special needs. *Developmental Psychology, 48*, 1476–1487. doi:10.1037/a0027537

Bitterman, A., Daley, T. C., Misra, S., Carlson, E., & Markowitz, J. (2008). A national sample of preschoolers with autism spectrum disorders: Special education services and parent satisfaction. *Journal of Autism and Developmental Disorders, 38*, 1509–1517. doi:10.1007/s10803-007-0531-9

Blacher, J., & Baker, B. L. (1994). Out-of-home placement for children with retardation: Family decision making and satisfaction. *Family Relations: Interdisciplinary Journal of Applied Family Studies, 43*, 10–15. doi:10.2307/585136

Blacher, J., & Baker, B. L. (2007). Positive impact of intellectual disability on families. *American Journal on Mental Retardation, 112*, 330–348. doi:10.1352/ 0895-8017(2007)112[0330:PIOIDO]2.0.CO;2

Blackorby, J., & Wagner, M. (1996). Longitudinal postschool outcomes of youth with disabilities: Findings from the National Longitudinal Transition Study.

Exceptional Children, 62, 399–413. Retrieved from http://www.cec.sped.org/content/NavigationMenu/Publications2/exceptionalchildren/

Blumberg, S. J., Read, D., Avila, R. M., & Bethell, C. D. (2010). Hispanic children with special health care needs in Spanish-language households. *Pediatrics, 126,* S120–S128. doi:10.1542/peds.2010-1466E

Boerner, K., Schulz, R., & Horowitz, A. (2004). Positive aspects of caregiving and adaptation to bereavement. *Psychology and Aging, 19,* 668–675. doi:10.1037/0882-7974. 19.4.668

Bonanno, G. A. (2004). Loss, trauma, and human resilience: Have we underestimated the human capacity to thrive after extremely adverse events? *American Psychologist, 59,* 20–28. doi:10.1037/0003-066X.59.1.20

Bonanno, G. A., Moskowitz, J. T., Papa, A., & Folkman, S. (2005). Resilience to loss in bereaved spouses, bereaved parents, and bereaved gay men. *Journal of Personality and Social Psychology, 88,* 827–843. doi:10.1037/0022-3514.88.5.827

Bonanno, G. A., Papa, A., Lalande, K., Westphal, M., & Coifman, K. (2004). The importance of being flexible: The ability to enhance and suppress emotional expression predicts long-term adjustment. *Psychological Science, 15,* 482–487. doi:10.1111/j.0956-7976.2004.00705.x

Bonanno, G. A., Wortman, C. B., Lehman, D. R., Tweed, R. G., Haring, M., Sonnega, J., & Nesse, R. M. (2002). Resilience to loss and chronic grief: A prospective study from preloss to 18-months postloss. *Journal of Personality and Social Psychology, 83,* 1150–1164. doi:10.1037/0022-3514.83.5.1150

Borthwick-Duffy, S. A. (1994). Epidemiology and prevalence of psychopathology in people with mental retardation. *Journal of Consulting and Clinical Psychology, 62,* 17–27. doi:10.1037/0022-006X.62.1.17

Boyle, C. A., Decoufle, P., & Yeargin-Allsopp, M. (1994). Prevalence and health impact of developmental disabilities in US children. *Pediatrics, 93,* 399–403. Retrieved from http://pediatrics.aappublications.org/content/93/3.toc

Braddock, D. L., & Parish, S. L. (2001). An institutional history of disability. In G. S. Albrecht, K. D. Seelman, & M. Bury (Eds.), *Handbook of disability studies* (pp. 11–68). Thousand Oaks, CA: Sage. doi:10.4135/9781412976251.n2

Bragiel, J., & Kaniok, P. E. (2011). Fathers' marital satisfaction and their involvement with their child with disabilities. *European Journal of Special Needs Education, 26,* 395–404. doi:10.1080/08856257.2011.595174

Bristol, M. M., Gallagher, J. J., & Holt, K. D. (1993). Maternal depressive symptoms in autism: Response to psychoeducational intervention. *Rehabilitation Psychology, 38,* 3–10. doi:10.1037/h0080290

Bristol, M. M., Gallagher, J. J., & Schopler, E. (1988). Mothers and fathers of young developmentally disabled and nondisabled boys: Adaptation and spousal support. *Developmental Psychology, 24,* 441–451. doi:10.1037/0012-1649.24.3.441

Bronfenbrenner, U. (1977). Toward an experimental ecology of human development. *American Psychologist, 32,* 513–531. doi:10.1037/0003-066X.32.7.513

Bronfenbrenner, U. (1999). Environments in developmental perspective: Theoretical and operational models. In S. L. Friedman & T. D. Wachs (Eds.), *Measuring environment across the life span: Emerging methods and concepts* (pp. 3–28). Washington, DC: American Psychological Association. doi:10.1037/10317-001

Bronfenbrenner, U., & Ceci, S. J. (1994). Nature-nurture reconceptualized in developmental perspective: A bioecological model. *Psychological Review, 101,* 568–586. doi:10.1037/0033-295X.101.4.568

Brown, R. I., Schalock, R. L., & Brown, I. (2009). Quality of life: Its application to persons with intellectual disabilities and their families—introduction and overview. *Journal of Policy and Practice in Intellectual Disabilities, 6,* 2–6. doi:10.1111/j.1741-1130.2008.00202.x

Browne, J. V., & Talmi, A. (2005). Family-based intervention to enhance infant–parent relationships in the neonatal intensive care unit. *Journal of Pediatric Psychology, 30,* 667–677. doi:10.1093/jpepsy/jsi053

Burke, M. M., Taylor, J. L., Urbano, R., & Hodapp, R. M. (2012). Predictors of future caregiving by adult siblings of individuals with intellectual and developmental disabilities. *American Journal on Intellectual and Developmental Disabilities, 117,* 33–47. doi:10.1352/1944-7558-117.1.33

Burton, C. M., & King, L. A. (2004). The health benefits of writing about intensely positive events. *Journal of Research in Personality, 38,* 150–163. doi:10.1016/S0092-6566(03)00058-8

Burton, C. M., & King, L. A. (2008). Effects of (very) brief writing on health: The two-minute miracle. *British Journal of Health Psychology, 13,* 9–14. doi:10.1348/135910707X250910

Byrne, P. S., & Long, B. (1976). *Doctors talking to patients: A study of verbal behaviours of doctors in the consultation.* London, England: Her Majesty's Stationery Office.

Cacioppo, J. T., Petty, R. E., Feinstein, J. A., & Jarvis, W. B. G. (1996). Dispositional differences in cognitive motivation: The life and times of individuals varying in need for cognition. *Psychological Bulletin, 119,* 197–253. doi:10.1037/0033-2909.119.2.197

Caldwell, J. (2008). Health and access to health care of female family caregivers of adults with developmental disabilities. *Journal of Disability Policy Studies, 19,* 68–79. doi:10.1177/1044207308316093

Calhoun, L. G., & Tedeschi, R. G. (2001). Posttraumatic growth: The positive lessons of loss. In R. A. Neimeyer (Ed.), *Meaning reconstruction and the experience of loss* (pp. 157–172). Washington, DC: American Psychological Association. doi:10.1037/10397-008

Callahan, J. L., & Hynan, M. T. (2002). Identifying mothers at risk for postnatal emotional distress: Further evidence for the validity of the perinatal posttraumatic stress disorder questionnaire. *Journal of Perinatology, 22,* 448–454. doi:10.1038/sj.jp.7210783

Callahan, K., Henson, R. K., & Cowan, A. K. (2008). Social validation of evidence-based practices in autism by parents, teachers, and administrators. *Journal of Autism and Developmental Disorders, 38,* 678–692. doi:10.1007/s10803-007-0434-9

Caravale, B., Tozzi, C., Albino, G., & Vicari, S. (2005). Cognitive development in low risk preterm infants at 3–4 years of life. *Archives of Disease in Childhood. Fetal and Neonatal Edition, 90,* F474–F479. doi:10.1136/adc.2004.070284

Carroll, D. W. (2008). Books written by parents of children with developmental disabilities: A quantitative text analysis. *Journal on Developmental Disabilities, 14*(3), 9–18. Retrieved from http://www.oadd.org/Published_Issues_142.html

Carroll, D. W. (2009). Cognitive and emotional language use in parents of children with developmental disabilities. *Journal on Developmental Disabilities, 15*(3), 88–95. Retrieved from http://www.oadd.org/Published_Issues_142.html

Carter, B. B., & Spencer, V. G. (2006). The fear factor: Bullying and students with disabilities. *International Journal of Special Education, 21*(1), 11–23. Retrieved from http://www.internationaljournalofspecialeducation.com/articles.cfm?y=2006&v=21&n=1

Cavet, J., & Sloper, P. (2004). Participation of disabled children in individual decisions about their lives and in public decisions about service development. *Children & Society, 18,* 278–290. doi:10.1002/chi.803

Ceci, S. J., & Hembrooke, H. A. (1995). A bioecological model of intellectual development. In P. Moen, G. H. Elder, Jr., & K. Luscher (Eds.), *Examining lives in context: Perspectives on the ecology of human development* (pp. 303–345). Washington, DC: American Psychological Association. doi:10.1037/10176-008

Centers for Disease Control and Prevention. (2012). Prevalence of autism spectrum disorders—Autism and Developmental Disabilities Monitoring Network, 14 Sites, United States, 2008. *Morbidity and Mortality Weekly Report. Surveillance Summaries, 61,* 1–19. Retrieved from http://www.cdc.gov/mmwr/preview/mmwrhtml/ss6103a1.htm?s_cid=ss6103a1_w

Charman, T., & Baird, G. (2002). Practitioner review: Diagnosis of autism spectrum disorder in 2- and 3-year-old children. *Journal of Child Psychology and Psychiatry, 43,* 289–305. doi:10.1111/1469-7610.00022

Chavira, V., Lopez, S. R., Blacher, J., & Shapiro, J. (2000). Latina mothers' attributions, emotions, and reactions to the problem behaviors of their children with developmental disabilities. *Journal of Child Psychology and Psychiatry, 41,* 245–252. doi:10.1111/1469-7610.00605

Clark, H. H. (1996). *Using language.* New York, NY: Cambridge University Press. doi:10.1017/CBO9780511620539

Coakley, R. M., Holmbeck, G. N., Friedman, D., Greenley, R. N., & Thill, A. W. (2002). A longitudinal study of pubertal timing, parent–child conflict, and cohesion in families of adolescents with spina bifida. *Journal of Pediatric Psychology, 27,* 461–473. doi:10.1093/jpepsy/27.5.461

Cole, B. A. (2005). "Good faith and effort?" Perspectives on educational inclusion. *Disability & Society, 20*, 331–344. doi:10.1080/09687590500060794

Cook, B. G., & Semmel, M. I. (1999). Peer acceptance of included students with disabilities as a function of severity of disability and classroom composition. *The Journal of Special Education, 33*, 50–61. doi:10.1177/002246699903300105

Cosden, M., Koegel, L. K., Koegel, R. L., Greenwell, A., & Klein, E. (2006). Strength-based assessment for children with autism spectrum disorder. *Research and Practice for Persons With Severe Disabilities, 31*, 134–143. Retrieved from http://www.ingentaconnect.com/content/tash/rpsd/2006/00000031/00000002/art00006

Crnic, K., Hoffman, C., Gaze, C., & Edelbrock, C. (2004). Understanding the emergence of behavior problems in young children with developmental delays. *Infants and Young Children, 17*, 223–235. doi:10.1097/00001163-200407000-00004

Crnic, K. A., Friedrich, W. N., & Greenberg, M. T. (1983). Adaptation of families with mentally retarded children: A model of stress, coping, and family ecology. *American Journal of Mental Deficiency, 88*, 125–138. Retrieved from http://psycnet.apa.org/psycinfo/1984-04250-001

Cummins, R. A. (2005). Moving from the quality of life concept to a theory. *Journal of Intellectual Disability Research, 49*, 699–706. doi:10.1111/j.1365-2788.2005.00738.x

Cunningham, S. D., Thomas, P. D., & Warschausky, S. (2007). Gender differences in peer relations of children with neurodevelopmental conditions. *Rehabilitation Psychology, 52*, 331–337. doi:10.1037/0090-5550.52.3.331

Cuskelly, M., & Gunn, P. (2003). Sibling relationships of children with Down syndrome: Perspectives of mothers, fathers, and siblings. *American Journal on Mental Retardation, 108*, 234–244. doi:10.1352/0895-8017(2003)108<234:SROCWD>2.0.CO;2

Cuskelly, M., Pulman, L., & Hayes, A. (1998). Parenting and employment decisions of parents with a preschool child with a disability. *Journal of Intellectual and Developmental Disability, 23*, 319–332. doi:10.1080/13668259800033801

Dale, E., Jahoda, A., & Knott, F. (2006). Mothers' attributions following their child's diagnosis of autism spectrum disorder: Exploring links with maternal levels of stress, depression, and expectations about their child's future. *Autism, 10*, 463–479. doi:10.1177/1362361306066600

Davies, R. (2005). Mothers' stories of loss: Their need to be with their dying child and their child's body after death. *Journal of Child Health Care, 9*, 288–300. doi:10.1177/1367493505056482

Davis, C. G., Wortman, C. B., Lehman, D. R., & Silver, R. C. (2000). Searching for meaning in loss: Are clinical assumptions correct? *Death Studies, 24*, 497–540. doi:10.1080/07481180050121471

Davis, J., & Watson, N. (2000). Disabled children's rights in every day life: Problematising notions of competency and promoting self-empowerment. *The International Journal of Children's Rights, 8*, 211–228. doi:10.1163/15718180020494622

Davis, N. O., & Carter, A. S. (2008). Parenting stress in mothers and fathers of toddlers with autism spectrum disorders: Associations with child characteristics. *Journal of Autism and Developmental Disorders, 38*, 1278–1291. doi:10.1007/s10803-007-0512-z

de Geeter, K. I., Poppes, P., & Vlaskamp, C. (2002). Parents as experts: The position of parents of children with profound multiple disabilities. *Child: Care, Health and Development, 28*, 443–453. doi:10.1046/j.1365-2214.2002.00294.x

DeGrace, B. W. (2004). The everyday occupation of families of children with autism. *American Journal of Occupational Therapy, 58*, 543–550. doi:10.5014/ajot.58.5.543

Deković, M., & Janssens, J. M. A. M. (1992). Parents' child-rearing style and child's sociometric status. *Developmental Psychology, 28*, 925–932. doi:10.1037/0012-1649.28.5.925

DeMier, R. L., Hynan, M. T., Hatfield, R. F., Varner, M. W., Harris, H. B., & Manniello, R. L. (2000). A measurement model of perinatal stressors: Identifying risk for postnatal emotional distress in mothers of high-risk infants. *Journal of Clinical Psychology, 56*, 89–100. doi:10.1002/(SICI)1097-4679(200001)56:1<89::AID-JCLP8>3.0.CO;2-6

Dempsey, I., & Keen, D. (2008). A review of processes and outcomes in family-centered services for children with a disability. *Topics in Early Childhood Special Education, 28*, 42–52. doi:10.1177/0271121408316699

Devlin, L., & Morrison, P. J. (2004). Accuracy of the clinical diagnosis of Down syndrome. *The Ulster Medical Journal, 73*(1), 4–12. Retrieved from http://www.ncbi.nlm.nih.gov/pmc/articles/PMC2475449/pdf/ulstermedj00003-0007.pdf

Diener, E., Emmons, R. A., Larson, R. J., & Griffin, S. (1985). The satisfaction with life scale. *Journal of Personality Assessment, 49*, 71–75. doi:10.1207/s15327752jpa4901_13

Doka, K. J., & Lavin, C. (2003). The paradox of ageing with developmental disabilities: Increasing needs, declining resources. *Ageing International, 28*, 135–154. doi:10.1007/s12126-003-1021-9

Drew, A., Baird, G., Baron-Cohen, S., Cox, A., Slonims, V., Wheelwright, S., . . . Charman, T. (2002). A pilot randomized control trial of a parent training intervention for pre-school children with autism. *European Child & Adolescent Psychiatry, 11*, 266–272. doi:10.1007/s00787-002-0299-6

Duckworth, A. L., Steen, T. A., & Seligman, M. E. P. (2005). Positive psychology in clinical practice. *Annual Review of Clinical Psychology, 1*, 629–651. doi:10.1146/annurev.clinpsy.1.102803.144154

Dunn, D. S. (2000). Social psychological issues in disability. In R. G. Frank & T. R. Elliott (Eds.), *Handbook of rehabilitation psychology* (pp. 565–584). Washington, DC: American Psychological Association. doi:10.1037/10361-027

Dweck, C. S., & Leggett, E. L. (1988). A social-cognitive approach to motivation and personality. *Psychological Review, 95*, 256–273. doi:10.1037/0033-295X.95.2.256

Dyson, L. L. (1997). Fathers and mothers of school-age children with developmental disabilities: Parental stress, family functioning, and social support. *American Journal on Mental Retardation, 102*, 267–279. doi:10.1352/0895-8017(1997)102<0267:FAMOSC>2.0.CO;2

Eakes, G. G., Burke, M. L., & Hainsworth, M. A. (1998). Middle-range theory of chronic sorrow. *Journal of Nursing Scholarship, 30*, 179–184. doi:10.1111/j.1547-5069.1998.tb01276.x

Education for all Handicapped Children Act of 1975, 20 U. S. C. 1401 et seq. Retrieved from http://www.eric.ed.gov/ERICWebPortal/search/detailmini.jsp?_nfpb=true&_&ERICExtSearch_SearchValue_0=ED140554&ERICExtSearch_SearchType_0=no&accno=ED140554

Ekas, N. V., Lickenbrock, D. M., & Whitman, T. L. (2010). Optimism, social support, and well-being in mothers of children with autism spectrum disorder. *Journal of Autism and Developmental Disorders, 40*, 1274–1284. doi:10.1007/s10803-010-0986-y

Elkins, J., van Kraayenoord, C. E., & Jobling, A. (2003). Parents' attitudes to inclusion of their children with special needs. *Journal of Research in Special Educational Needs, 3*, 122–129. doi:10.1111/1471-3802.00005

Emmons, R. A., & McCullough, M. E. (2003). Counting blessings versus burdens: An experimental investigation of gratitude and subjective well-being in daily life. *Journal of Personality and Social Psychology, 84*, 377–389. doi:10.1037/0022-3514.84.2.377

Erwin, E. J., & Soodak, L. C. (1995). I never knew I could stand up to the system: Families' perspectives on pursuing inclusive education. *Journal of the Association for Persons with Severe Handicaps, 20*, 136–146. Retrieved from http://psycnet.apa.org/psycinfo/1996-18503-001

Esbensen, A. J., Bishop, S., Seltzer, M. M., Greenberg, J. S., & Taylor, J. L. (2010). Comparisons between individuals with autism spectrum disorders and individuals with Down syndrome in adulthood. *American Journal on Intellectual and Developmental Disabilities, 115*, 277–290. doi:10.1352/1944-7558-115.4.277

Essex, E. L., Seltzer, M. M., & Krauss, M. W. (1997). Residential transitions of adults with mental retardation: Predictors of waiting list use and placement. *American Journal on Mental Retardation, 101*, 613–629. Retrieved from http://www.ncbi.nlm.nih.gov/pubmed/9152476

Essner, B. S., & Holmbeck, G. N. (2010). The impact of family, peer, and school contexts on depressive symptoms in adolescents with spina bifida. *Rehabilitation Psychology, 55*, 340–350. doi:10.1037/a0021664

Favazza, P. C., Phillipsen, L., & Kumar, P. (2000). Measuring and promoting acceptance of young children with disabilities. *Exceptional Children, 66*, 491–508. Retrieved from http://www.cec.sped.org/content/NavigationMenu/Publications2/exceptionalchildren/

Featherstone, H. (1981). *A difference in the family: Living with a disabled child.* New York, NY: Penguin.

Feldman, M., McDonald, L., Serbin, L., Stack, D., Secco, M. L., & Yu, C. T. (2007). Predictors of depressive symptoms in primary caregivers of young children with or at risk for developmental delay. *Journal of Intellectual Disability Research, 51*, 606–619. doi:10.1111/j.1365-2788.2006.00941.x

Feldman, M. A., & Werner, S. E. (2002). Collateral effects of behavioral parent training on families of children with developmental disabilities and behavior disorders. *Behavioral Interventions, 17*, 75–83. doi:10.1002/bin.111

Fiese, B. H., Tomcho, T. J., Douglas, M., Josephs, K., Poltrock, S., & Baker, T. (2002). A review of 50 years of research on naturally occurring family routines and rituals: Cause for celebration? *Journal of Family Psychology, 16*, 381–390. doi:10.1037/0893-3200.16.4.381

Fisman, S., Wolf, L., Ellison, D., & Freeman, T. (2000). A longitudinal study of siblings of children with chronic disabilities. *Canadian Journal of Psychiatry/La Revue canadienne de psychiatrie, 45*, 369–375. Retrieved from http://psycnet.apa.org/psycinfo/2000-07768-005

Fisman, S. N., Wolf, L. C., & Noh, S. (1989). Marital intimacy in parents of exceptional children. *Canadian Journal of Psychiatry/La Revue canadienne de psychiatrie, 34*, 519–525. Retrieved from http://www.ncbi.nlm.nih.gov/pubmed/2527593

Flannery, K. B., Yovanoff, P., Benz, M. R., & Kato, M. M. (2008). Improving employment outcomes of individuals with disabilities through short-term training. *Career Development for Exceptional Individuals, 31*, 26–36. doi:10.1177/0885728807313779

Fleischmann, A. (2005). The hero's story and autism: Grounded theory study of websites for parents of children with autism. *Autism, 9*, 299–316. doi:10.1177/1362361305054410

Florian, V., & Findler, L. (2001). Mental health and marital adaptation among mothers of children with cerebral palsy. *American Journal of Orthopsychiatry, 71*, 358–367. doi:10.1037/0002-9432.71.3.358

Floyd, F. J., & Gallagher, E. M. (1997). Parental stress, care demands, and use of support services for school-age children with disabilities and behavior problems. *Family Relations, 46*, 359–371. doi:10.2307/585096

Folkman, S., & Moskowitz, J. T. (2000). Positive affect and the other side of coping. *American Psychologist, 55*, 647–654. doi:10.1037/0003-066X.55.6.647

Fombonne, E. (2003). Epidemiological surveys of autism and other pervasive developmental disorders: An update. *Journal of Autism and Developmental Disorders, 33*, 365–382. doi:10.1023/A:1025054610557

Fombonne, E., Zakarian, R., Bennett, A., Meng, L., & McLean-Heywood, D. (2006). Pervasive developmental disorders in Montreal, Quebec, Canada: Prevalence and links with immunizations. *Pediatrics, 118*, e139–e150. doi:10.1542/peds.2005-2993

Fordyce, M. W. (1977). Development of a program to increase personal happiness. *Journal of Counseling Psychology, 24*, 511–521. doi:10.1037/0022-0167.24.6.511

Fordyce, M. W. (1983). A program to increase happiness: Further studies. *Journal of Counseling Psychology, 30,* 483–498. doi:10.1037/0022-0167.30.4.483

Fountain, C., King, M. D., & Bearman, P. S. (2011). Age of diagnosis for autism: Individual and community factors across 10 birth cohorts. *Journal of Epidemiology and Community Health, 65,* 503–510. doi:10.1136/jech.2009.104588

Fox, L., Vaughn, B. J., Wyatte, M. L., & Dunlap, G. (2002). "We can't expect other people to understand": Family perspectives on problem behavior. *Exceptional Children, 68,* 437–450. Retrieved from http://cec.metapress.com/content/r471 68175572/?p=76b3b6e063134978859b73cdd302e829&pi=39

Frankland, H. C., Turnbull, A. P., Wehmeyer, M. L., & Blackmountain, L. (2004). An exploration of the self-determination construct and disability as it relates to the Diné (Navajo) culture. *Education and Training in Developmental Disabilities, 39,* 191–205.

Franklin, A., & Sloper, P. (2009). Supporting the participation of disabled children and young people in decision-making. *Children & Society, 23,* 3–15. doi:10.1111/j.1099-0860.2007.00131.x

Frantz, T. T., Farrell, M. M., & Trolley, B. C. (2001). Positive outcomes of losing a loved one. In R. A. Neimeyer (Ed.), *Meaning reconstruction & the experience of loss* (pp. 191–209). Washington, DC: American Psychological Association. doi:10.1037/10397-010

Frazier, P., Tennen, H., Gavian, M., Park, C., Tomich, P., & Tashiro, T. (2009). Does self-reported posttraumatic growth reflect genuine positive change? *Psychological Science, 20,* 912–919. doi:10.1111/j.1467-9280.2009.02381.x

Frederickson, N. L., & Furnham, A. F. (1998). Sociometric-status-group classification of mainstreamed children who have moderate learning difficulties: An investigation of personal and environmental factors. *Journal of Educational Psychology, 90,* 772–783. doi:10.1037/0022-0663.90.4.772

Fredrickson, B. L. (1998). What good are positive emotions? *Review of General Psychology, 2,* 300–319. doi:10.1037/1089-2680.2.3.300

Fredrickson, B. L., & Branigan, C. (2005). Positive emotions broaden the scope of attention and thought–action repertoires. *Cognition and Emotion, 19,* 313–332. doi:10.1080/02699930441000238

Fredrickson, B. L., Mancuso, R. A., Branigan, C., & Tugade, M. M. (2000). The undoing effect of positive emotions. *Motivation and Emotion, 24,* 237–258. doi:10.1023/A:1010796329158

Freedman, R. I., Griffiths, D., Krauss, M. W., & Seltzer, M. M. (1999). Patterns of respite use by aging mothers of adults with mental retardation. *Mental Retardation, 37,* 93–103. doi:http://dx.doi.org/10.1352/00476765(1999)037<0093:PO RUBA>2.0.CO;2

Freedman, R. I., Krauss, M. W., & Seltzer, M. M. (1997). Aging parents' residential plans for adult children with mental retardation. *Mental Retardation, 35,* 114–123. doi:10.1352/0047-6765(1997)035<0114:APRPFA>2.0.CO;2

Freedman, S. R., & Enright, R. D. (1996). Forgiveness as an intervention goal with incest survivors. *Journal of Consulting and Clinical Psychology, 64,* 983–992. doi:10.1037/0022-006X.64.5.983

Friedman, D., Holmbeck, G. N., DeLucia, C., Jandasek, B., & Zebracki, K. (2009). Trajectories of autonomy development across the adolescent transition in children with spina bifida. *Rehabilitation Psychology, 54,* 16–27. doi:10.1037/a0014279

Galatzer-Levy, I. R., Mazursky, H., Mancini, A. D., & Bonanno, G. A. (2011). What we don't expect when expecting: Evidence for heterogeneity in subjective well-being in response to parenthood. *Journal of Family Psychology, 25,* 384–392. doi:10.1037/a0023759

Galil, A., Bachner, Y. G., Merrick, J., Flusser, H., Lubetzky, H., Helman, N., & Carmel, S. (2006). Physician–parent communication as predictor of parent satisfaction with child development services. *Research in Developmental Disabilities, 27,* 233–242. doi:10.1016/j.ridd.2005.03.004

Garel, M., Dardennes, M., & Blondel, B. (2007). Mothers' psychological distress 1 year after preterm childbirth. Results of the epipage qualitative study. *Child: Care, Health and Development, 33,* 137–143. doi:10.1111/j.1365-2214.2006.00663.x

Garland, R. (2010). *The eye of the beholder: Deformity and disability in the Graeco-Roman world* (2nd ed.). London, England: Bristol Classical Press.

Garth, B., Murphy, G. C., & Reddihough, D. S. (2009). Perceptions of participation: Child patients with a disability in the doctor–patient–child partnership. *Patient Education and Counseling, 74,* 45–52. doi:10.1016/j.pec.2008.07.031

Gernsbacher, M. A., Dawson, M., & Goldsmith, H. H. (2005). Three reasons not to believe in an autism epidemic. *Current Directions in Psychological Science, 14,* 55–58. doi:10.1111/j.0963-7214.2005.00334.x

Gill, J., & Liamputtong, P. (2011). Being the mother of a child with Asperger's syndrome: Women's experience of stigma. *Health Care for Women International, 32,* 708–722. doi:10.1080/07399332.2011.555830

Gill, V. T., & Maynard, D. W. (1995). On "labeling" in actual interaction: Delivering and receiving diagnoses of developmental disabilities. *Social Problems, 42,* 11–37. doi:10.2307/3097003

Gillham, J. E., Shatte, A. J., Reivich, K. J., & Seligman, M. E. P. (2001). Optimism, pessimism, and explanatory style. In E. C. Chang (Ed.), *Optimism and pessimism: Implications for theory, research, and practice* (pp. 53–75). Washington, DC: American Psychological Association. doi:10.1037/10385-003

Gilmore, L., Campbell, J., & Cuskelly, M. (2003). Developmental expectations, personality stereotypes, and attitudes toward inclusive education: Community and teacher views of Down syndrome. *International Journal of Disability, Development and Education, 50,* 65–76. doi:10.1080/1034912032000053340

Glidden, L. M., & Jobe, B. M. (2006). The longitudinal course of depression in adoptive and birth mothers of children with intellectual disabilities.

Journal of Policy and Practice in Intellectual Disabilities, 3, 139–142. doi:10.1111/j.1741-1130.2006.00067.x

Glidden, L. M., & Schoolcraft, S. A. (2003). Depression: Its trajectory and correlates in mothers rearing children with intellectual disability. *Journal of Intellectual Disability Research, 47,* 250–263. doi:10.1046/j.1365-2788.2003.00487.x

Glück, J., Bluck, S., Baron, J., & McAdams, D. P. (2005). The wisdom of experience: Autobiographical narratives across adulthood. *International Journal of Behavioral Development, 29,* 197–208. doi:10.1177/01650250444000504

Goffman, E. (1963). *Stigma: Notes on the management of spoiled identity.* New York, NY: Simon and Schuster.

Goin-Kochel, R. P., Mackintosh, V. H., & Myers, B. J. (2006). How many doctors does it take to make an autism spectrum diagnosis? *Autism, 10,* 439–451. doi:10.1177/1362361306066601

Goldberg, S., Marcovitch, S., MacGregor, D., & Lojkasek, M. (1986). Family responses to developmentally delayed preschoolers: Etiology and the father's role. *American Journal of Mental Deficiency, 90,* 610–617. Retrieved from http://psycnet.apa.org/psycinfo/1986-24587-001

Goodey, C. F. (2001). What is developmental disability? The origin and nature of our conceptual models. *Journal on Developmental Disabilities, 8,* 1–18. Retrieved from http://www.oadd.org/Published_Issues_142.html

Graungaard, A. H., Andersen, J. S., & Skov, L. (2011). When resources get sparse: A longitudinal, qualitative study of emotions, coping and resource-creation when parenting a young child with severe disabilities. *Health, 15,* 115–136. doi:10.1177/1363459309360794

Graungaard, A. H., & Skov, L. (2007). Why do we need a diagnosis? A qualitative study of parents' experiences, coping and needs, when the newborn child is severely disabled. *Child: Care, Health and Development, 33,* 296–307. doi:10.1111/j.1365-2214.2006.00666.x

Gray, D. (2002). Ten years on: A longitudinal study of families with autism. *Journal of Intellectual and Developmental Disability, 27,* 215–222. doi:10.1080/1366825021000008639

Gray, S. (2009). Happy ending, complicated beginning. In D. Meyer (Ed.), *Thicker than water: Essays by adult siblings of people with disabilities* (pp. 117–122). Bethesda, MD: Woodbine House.

Green, S. E. (2001). "Oh, those therapists will become your best friends": Maternal satisfaction with clinics providing physical, occupational, and speech therapy services to children with disabilities. *Sociology of Health & Illness, 23,* 798–828. doi:10.1111/1467-9566.00276

Green, S. E. (2002). Mothering Amanda: Musings on the experience of raising a child with cerebral palsy. *Journal of Loss and Trauma, 7,* 21–34. doi:10.1080/108114402753344463

Green, S. E. (2007). "We're tired, not sad": Benefits and burdens of mothering a child with a disability. *Social Science & Medicine, 64,* 150–163. doi:10.1016/j.socscimed.2006.08.025

Greenberg, J. S., Seltzer, M. M., & Greenley, J. R. (1993). Aging parents of adults with disabilities: The gratifications and frustrations of later-life caregiving. *The Gerontologist, 33,* 542–550. doi:10.1093/geront/33.4.542

Greenberg, J. S., Seltzer, M. M., Hong, J., & Orsmond, G. I. (2006). Bidirectional effects of expressed emotion and behavior problems and symptoms in adolescents and adults with autism. *American Journal on Mental Retardation, 111,* 229–249. doi:10.1352/0895-8017(2006)111[229:BEOEEA]2.0.CO;2

Greenberg, J. S., Seltzer, M. M., Orsmond, G. I., & Krauss, M. W. (1999). Siblings of adults with mental illness or mental retardation: Current involvement and expectation of future caregiving. *Psychiatric Services, 50,* 1214–1219. Retrieved from http://ps.psychiatryonline.org/Issue.aspx?issueID=3523&direction=P&journalID=18

Greenley, R. N., Coakley, R. M., Holmbeck, G. N., Jandasek, B., & Wills, K. (2006). Condition-related knowledge among children with spina bifida: Longitudinal changes and predictors. *Journal of Pediatric Psychology, 31,* 828–839. doi:10.1093/jpepsy/jsj097

Grossman, P., Tiefenthaler-Gilmer, U., Raysz, A., & Kesper, U. (2007). Mindfulness training as an intervention for fibromyalgia: Evidence of postintervention and 3-year follow-up benefits in well-being. *Psychotherapy and Psychosomatics, 76,* 226–233. doi:10.1159/000101501

Gundersen, T. (2011). "One wants to know what a chromosome is": The internet as a coping resource when adjusting to life parenting a child with a rare genetic disorder. *Sociology of Health & Illness, 33,* 81–95. doi:10.1111/j.1467-9566.2010.01277.x

Gupta, S., & Bonanno, G. A. (2011). Complicated grief and deficits in emotional expressive flexibility. *Journal of Abnormal Psychology, 120,* 635–643. doi:10.1037/a0023541

Guralnick, M. J. (1999). Family and child influences on the peer-related social competence of children with developmental delays. *Mental Retardation and Developmental Disabilities Research Reviews, 5,* 21–29. doi:10.1002/(SICI)1098-2779(1999)5:1<21::AID-MRDD3>3.0.CO;2-O

Guralnick, M. J. (2004). Family investments in response to the developmental challenges of young children with disabilities. In A. Kalil & T. Deleire (Eds.), *Family investments in children's potential: Resources and parenting behaviors that promote success* (pp. 119–137). Mahwah, NJ: Lawrence Erlbaum.

Guralnick, M. J., Connor, R. T., Neville, B., & Hammond, M. A. (2006). Promoting the peer-related social development of young children with mild developmental delays: Effectiveness of a comprehensive intervention. *American Journal on Mental Retardation, 111,* 336–356. doi:10.1352/0895-8017(2006)111[336:PTPSDO]2.0.CO;2

Guralnick, M. J., Neville, B., Connor, R. T., & Hammond, M. A. (2003). Family factors associated with the peer social competence of young children with mild delays. *American Journal on Mental Retardation, 108,* 272–287. doi:10.1352/0895-8017(2003)108<272:FFAWTP>2.0.CO;2

Guralnick, M. J., Neville, B., Hammond, M. A., & Connor, R. T. (2007). Linkages between delayed children's social interactions with mothers and peers. *Child Development, 78,* 459–473. doi:10.1111/j.1467-8624.2007.01009.x

Ha, J.-H., Hong, J., Seltzer, M. M., & Greenberg, J. S. (2008). Age and gender differences in the well-being of parents with children with mental health or developmental problems: Report of a national study. *Journal of Health and Social Behavior, 49,* 301–316. doi:10.1177/002214650804900305

Hannah, M. E., & Midlarsky, E. (2005). Helping by siblings of children with mental retardation. *American Journal on Mental Retardation, 110,* 87–99. doi:10.1352/0895-8017(2005)110<87:HBSOCW>2.0.CO;2

Harris, J. C. (2010). *Intellectual disability: A guide for families and professionals.* New York, NY: Oxford University Press.

Harry, B. (2008). Collaboration with culturally and linguistically diverse families: Ideal versus reality. *Exceptional Children, 74,* 372–388.

Hartley, S. L., Barker, E. T., Seltzer, M. M., Floyd, F., Greenberg, J., Orsmond, G., . . . Bolt, D. (2010). The relative risk and timing of divorce in families of children with an autism spectrum disorder. *Journal of Family Psychology, 24,* 449–457. doi:10.1037/a0019847

Hartley, S. L., Barker, E. T., Seltzer, M. M., Greenberg, J. S., & Floyd, F. J. (2011). Marital satisfaction and parenting experiences of mothers and fathers of adolescents and adults with autism. *American Journal on Intellectual and Developmental Disabilities, 116,* 81–95. doi:10.1352/1944-7558-116.1.81

Hartshorne, T. S. (2002). Mistaking courage for denial: Family resilience after the birth of a child with severe disabilities. *The Journal of Individual Psychology, 58,* 263–278. Retrieved from http://psycnet.apa.org/psycinfo/2002-04435-007

Hastings, R. P. (1997). Grandparents of children with disabilities: A review. *International Journal of Disability, Development and Education, 44,* 329–340. doi:10.1080/0156655970440404

Hastings, R. P. (2003a). Behavioral adjustment of siblings of children with autism engaged in applied behavior analysis early intervention programs: The moderating role of social support. *Journal of Autism and Developmental Disorders, 33,* 141–150. doi:10.1023/A:1022983209004

Hastings, R. P. (2003b). Child behaviour problems and partner mental health as correlates of stress in mothers and fathers of children with autism. *Journal of Intellectual Disability Research, 47,* 231–237. doi:10.1046/j.1365-2788.2003.00485.x

Hastings, R. P., & Beck, A. (2004). Practitioner review: Stress intervention for parents of children with intellectual disabilities. *Journal of Child Psychology and Psychiatry, 45,* 1338–1349. doi:10.1111/j.1469-7610.2004.00357.x

Hastings, R. P., Beck, A., & Hill, C. (2005). Positive contributions made by children with an intellectual disability in the family: Mothers' and fathers' perceptions. *Journal of Intellectual Disabilities, 9*, 155–165. doi:10.1177/1744629505053930

Hastings, R. P., Daley, D., Burns, C., & Beck, A. (2006). Maternal distress and expressed emotion: Cross-sectional and longitudinal relationships with behavior problems of children with intellectual disabilities. *American Journal on Mental Retardation, 111*, 48–61. doi:10.1352/0895-8017(2006)111[48:MDAEEC]2.0.CO;2

Hastings, R. P., & Lloyd, T. (2007). Expressed emotion in families of children and adults with intellectual disabilities. *Mental Retardation and Developmental Disabilities Research Reviews, 13*, 339–345. doi:10.1002/mrdd.20173

Hastings, R. P., & Taunt, H. M. (2002). Positive perceptions in families of children with developmental disabilities. *American Journal on Mental Retardation, 107*, 116–127. doi:10.1352/0895-8017(2002)107<0116:PPIFOC>2.0.CO;2

Hastings, R. P., Thomas, H., & Delwiche, N. (2002). Grandparent support for families of children with Down's syndrome. *Journal of Applied Research in Intellectual Disabilities, 15*, 97–104. doi:10.1046/j.1360 2322.2001.00097.x

Hatton, C., Emerson, E., Graham, H., Blacher, J., & Llewellyn, G. (2010). Changes in family composition and marital status in families with a young child with cognitive delay. *Journal of Applied Research in Intellectual Disabilities, 23*, 14–26. doi:10.1111/j.1468-3148.2009.00543.x

Heath, C. (1992). The delivery and reception of diagnosis in the general-practice consultation. In P. Drew & J. Heritage (Eds.), *Talk at work: Interaction in institutional settings* (pp. 235–267). Cambridge: Cambridge University Press.

Heiman, T. (2002). Parents of children with disabilities: Resilience, coping, and future expectations. *Journal of Developmental and Physical Disabilities, 14*, 159–171. doi:10.1023/A:1015219514621

Helgeson, V. S., Reynolds, K. A., & Tomich, P. L. (2006). A meta-analytic review of benefit finding and growth. *Journal of Consulting and Clinical Psychology, 74*, 797–816. doi:10.1037/0022-006X.74.5.797

Heritage, J. (2005). Conversation analysis and institutional talk. In R. Sanders & K. Fitch (Eds.), *Handbook of language and social interaction* (pp. 103–147). Mahwah, NJ: Erlbaum.

Heritage, J., & Maynard, D. W. (2006). Problems and prospects in the study of physician-patient interaction: 30 years of research. *Annual Review of Sociology, 32*, 351–374. doi:10.1146/annurev.soc.32.082905.093959

Heritage, J., & Robinson, J. D. (2006). The structure of patients' presenting concerns: Physicians' opening questions. *Health Communication, 19*, 89–102. doi:10.1207/s15327027hc1902_1

Heritage, J., Robinson, J. D., Elliott, M. N., Beckett, M., & Wilkes, M. (2007). Reducing patients' unmet concerns in primary care: The difference one word can make. *Journal of General Internal Medicine, 22*, 1429–1433. doi:10.1007/s11606-007-0279-0

Hillman, J. (2007). Grandparents of children with autism: A review with recommendations for education, practice, and policy. *Educational Gerontology, 33,* 513–527. doi:10.1080/03601270701328425

Hodapp, R. M., Ly, T. M., Fidler, D. J., & Ricci, L. A. (2001). Less stress, more rewarding: Parenting children with Down syndrome. *Parenting: Science and Practice, 1,* 317–337. doi:10.1207/S15327922PAR0104_3

Holditch-Davis, D., Bartlett, T. R., Blickman, A. L., & Miles, M. S. (2003). Posttraumatic stress symptoms in mothers of premature infants. *Journal of Obstetric, Gynecologic, and Neonatal Nursing, 32,* 161–171. doi:10.1177/0884217503252035

Holditch-Davis, D., Miles, M. S., Weaver, M. A., Black, B., Beeber, L., Thoyre, S., & Engelke, S. (2009). Patterns of distress in African American mothers of preterm infants. *Journal of Developmental and Behavioral Pediatrics, 30,* 193–205. doi:10.1097/DBP.0b013e3181a7ee53

Holmbeck, G. N., DeLucia, C., Essner, B., Kelly, L., Zebracki, K., Friedman, D., & Jandasek, B. (2010). Trajectories of psychosocial adjustment in adolescents with spina bifida: A 6-year, four-wave longitudinal follow-up. *Journal of Consulting and Clinical Psychology, 78,* 511–525. doi:10.1037/a0019599

Holmbeck, G. N., & Devine, K. A. (2010). Psychosocial and family functioning in spina bifida. *Developmental Disabilities Research Reviews, 16,* 40–46. doi:10.1002/ddrr.90

Holmbeck, G. N., Johnson, S. Z., Wills, K. E., McKernon, W., Rose, B., Erklin, S., & Kemper, T. (2002). Observed and perceived parental overprotection in relation to psychosocial adjustment in preadolescents with a physical disability: The mediational role of behavioral autonomy. *Journal of Consulting and Clinical Psychology, 70,* 96–110. doi:10.1037/0022-006X.70.1.96

Holmbeck, G. N., Westhoven, V. C., Phillips, W. S., Bowers, R., Gruse, C., Nikolopoulos, T., . . . Davison, K. (2003). A multimethod, multi-informant, and multidimensional perspective on psychosocial adjustment in preadolescents with spina bifida. *Journal of Consulting and Clinical Psychology, 71,* 782–796. doi:10.1037/0022-006X.71.4.782

Holzheimer, L., Mohay, H., & Masters, I. B. (1998). Educating young children about asthma: Comparing the effectiveness of a developmentally appropriate asthma education video tape and picture book. *Child: Care, Health and Development, 24,* 85–99. doi:10.1046/j.1365-2214.1998.00055.x

Hooley, J. M., & Gotlib, I. H. (2000). A diathesis–stress conceptualization of expressed emotion and clinical outcome. *Applied & Preventive Psychology, 9,* 135–151. doi:10.1016/S0962-1849(05)80001-0

Hudson, A. M., Matthews, J. M., Gavidia-Payne, S. T., Cameron, C. A., Mildon, R. L., Radler, G. A., & Nankervis, K. L. (2003). Evaluation of an intervention system for parents of children with intellectual disability and challenging behaviour. *Journal of Intellectual Disability Research, 47,* 238–249. doi:10.1046/j.1365-2788.2003.00486.x

Ingersoll, B., & Hambrick, D. Z. (2011). The relationship between the broader autism phenotype, child severity, and stress and depression in parents of children with autism spectrum disorders. *Research in Autism Spectrum Disorders, 5,* 337–344. doi:10.1016/j.rasd.2010.04.017

Ingersoll, B., Meyer, K., & Becker, M. W. (2011). Increased rates of depressed mood in mothers of children with ASD associated with the presence of the broader autism phenotype. *Autism Research, 4,* 143–148. doi:10.1002/aur.170

Isaacs, B. J., Brown, I., Brown, R. I., Baum, N., Myerscough, T., Neikrug, S., . . . Wang, M. (2007). The international family quality of life project: Goals and description of a survey tool. *Journal of Policy and Practice in Intellectual Disabilities, 4,* 177–185. doi:10.1111/j.1741-1130.2007.00116.x

Jang, S. J., & Appelbaum, E. (2010). Work–life balance in extraordinary circumstances. *Journal of Women, Politics & Policy, 31,* 313–333. doi:10.1080/15544 77X.2010.517156

Javier, J. R., Huffman, L. C., Mendoza, F. S., & Wise, P. H. (2010). Children with special health care needs: How immigrant status is related to health care access, health care utilization, and health status. *Maternal and Child Health Journal, 14,* 567–579. doi:10.1007/s10995-009-0487-9

Johnson, K. J., Waugh, C. E., & Fredrickson, B. L. (2010). Smile to see the forest: Facially expressed positive emotions broaden cognition. *Cognition and Emotion, 24,* 299–321. doi:10.1080/02699930903384667

Johnston, C., Hessl, D., Blasey, C., Eliez, S., Erba, H., Dyer-Friedman, J., . . . Reiss, A. L. (2003). Factors associated with parenting stress in mothers of children with fragile X syndrome. *Journal of Developmental and Behavioral Pediatrics, 24,* 267–275. doi:10.1097/00004703-200308000-00008

Jotzo, M., & Poets, C. F. (2005). Helping parents cope with the trauma of premature birth: An evaluation of a trauma-preventive psychological intervention. *Pediatrics, 115,* 915–919. doi:10.1542/peds.2004-0370

Jung, A. W. (2011). Individualized education programs (IEPs) and barriers for parents from culturally and linguistically diverse backgrounds. *Multicultural Education, 18,* 21–25.

Kagan, C., Lewis, S., Heaton, P., & Cranshaw, M. (1999). Enabled or disabled? Working parents of disabled children and the provision of child-care. *Journal of Community & Applied Social Psychology, 9,* 369–381. doi:10.1002/(SICI)1099-1298(199909/10)9:5<369::AID-CASP527>3.0.CO;2-H

Kaminsky, L., & Dewey, D. (2001). Siblings relationships of children with autism. *Journal of Autism and Developmental Disorders, 31,* 399–410. doi:10.1023/A:1010664603039

Kasari, C., Freeman, S. F. N., Bauminger, N., & Alkin, M. C. (1999). Parental perspectives on inclusion: Effects of autism and Down syndrome. *Journal of Autism and Developmental Disorders, 29,* 297–305. doi:10.1023/A:1022159302571

Katz, R. T. (2003). Life expectancy for children with cerebral palsy and mental retar-dation: Implications for life care planning. *NeuroRehabilitation, 18*, 261–270. Retrieved from http://iospress.metapress.com/content/g4tfh0mrp33x/?p=d2baf 5d7bb454bdb9f7c507a8e7c698e&pi=52

Katz, S., & Kessel, L. (2002). Grandparents of children with developmental disabili-ties: Perceptions, beliefs, and involvement in their care. *Issues in Comprehensive Pediatric Nursing, 25*, 113–128. doi:10.1080/01460860290042530

Kausar, S., Jevne, R. F., & Sobsey, D. (2003). Hope in families of children with developmental disabilities. *Journal on Developmental Disabilities, 10*, 35–46. Retrieved from http://www.oadd.org/Published_Issues_142.html

Kayfitz, A. D., Gragg, M. N., & Orr, R. R. (2010). Positive experiences of mothers and fathers of children with autism. *Journal of Applied Research in Intellectual Disabilities, 23*, 337–343. doi:10.1111/j.1468-3148.2009.00539.x

Kearney, P. M., & Griffin, T. (2001). Between joy and sorrow: Being a parent of a child with developmental disability. *Journal of Advanced Nursing, 34*, 582–592. doi:10.1046/j.1365-2648.2001.01787.x

Kelly, L. M., Zebracki, K., Holmbeck, G. N., & Gershenson, L. (2008). Adoles-cent development and family functioning in youth with spina bifida. *Journal of Pediatric Rehabilitation Medicine, 1*, 291–302. Retrieved from http://iospress. metapress.com/content/r7413q317242/?p=87b04ded4b2d467c824c90a17c8bf8 d7&pi=12

Keogh, B. K., Garnier, H. E., Bernheimer, L. P., & Gallimore, R. (2000). Models of child–family interactions for children with developmental delays: Child-driven or transactional? *American Journal on Mental Retardation, 105*, 32–46. doi:10.1352/0895-8017(2000)105<0032:MOCIFC>2.0.CO;2

Kersh, J., Hedvat, T. T., Hauser-Cram, P., & Warfield, M. E. (2006). The contri-bution of marital quality to the well-being of parents of children with devel-opmental disabilities. *Journal of Intellectual Disability Research, 50*, 883–893. doi:10.1111/j.1365-2788.2006.00906.x

King, G., Baxter, D., Rosenbaum, P., Zwaigenbaum, L., & Bates, A. (2009). Belief sys-tems of families of children with autism spectrum disorders or Down syndrome. *Focus on Autism and Other Developmental Disabilities, 24*, 50–64. doi:10.1177/ 1088357608329173

King, G., King, S., Rosenbaum, P., & Goffin, R. (1999). Family-centered caregiving and well-being of parents of children with disabilities: Linking process with outcomes. *Journal of Pediatric Psychology, 24*, 41–53. doi:10.1093/jpepsy/24.1.41

King, G. A., Baldwin, P. J., Currie, M., & Evans, J. (2005). Planning successful tran-sitions from school to adult roles for youth with disabilities. *Children's Health Care, 34*, 193–216. doi:10.1207/s15326888chc3403_3

King, G. A., Zwaigenbaum, L., King, S., Baxter, D., Rosenbaum, P., & Bates, A. (2006). A qualitative investigation of changes in the belief systems of families of children with autism or Down syndrome. *Child: Care, Health and Development, 32*, 353–369. doi:10.1111/j.1365-2214.2006.00571.x

King, L. A., & Hicks, J. A. (2006). Narrating the self in the past and the future: Implications for maturity. *Research in Human Development, 3*, 121–138. doi:10.1080/15427609.2006.9683365

King, L. A., Hicks, J. A., Krull, J. L., & Del Gaiso, A. K. (2006). Positive affect and the experience of meaning in life. *Journal of Personality and Social Psychology, 90*, 179–196. doi:10.1037/0022-3514.90.1.179

King, L. A., & Patterson, C. (2000). Reconstructing life goals after the birth of a child with Down syndrome: Finding happiness and growing. *International Journal of Rehabilitation and Health, 5*, 17–30. doi:10.1023/A:1012955018489

King, L. A., & Raspin, C. (2004). Lost and found possible selves, subjective well-being, and ego development in divorced women. *Journal of Personality, 72*, 603–632. doi:10.1111/j.0022-3506.2004.00274.x

King, L. A., Scollon, C. K., Ramsey, C., & Williams, T. (2000). Stories of life transition: Subjective well-being and ego development in parents of children with Down syndrome. *Journal of Research in Personality, 34*, 509–536. doi:10.1006/jrpe.2000.2285

King, L. A., & Smith, N. G. (2004). Gay and straight possible selves: Goals, identity, subjective well-being, and personality development. *Journal of Personality, 72*, 967–994. doi:10.1111/j.0022-3506.2004.00287.x

King, M., & Bearman, P. (2009). Diagnostic change and the increased prevalence of autism. *International Journal of Epidemiology, 38*, 1224–1234. doi:10.1093/ije/dyp261

King, S., Teplicky, R., King, G., & Rosenbaum, P. (2004). Family-centered service for children with cerebral palsy and their families: A review of the literature. *Seminars in Pediatric Neurology, 11*, 78–86. doi:10.1016/j.spen.2004.01.009

Kirkham, M. A. (1993). Two-year follow-up of skills training with mothers of children with disabilities. *American Journal on Mental Retardation, 97*, 509–520. Retrieved from http://psycnet.apa.org/psycinfo/1993-26647-001

Kitchin, R. (1998). "Out of place", "knowing one's place": Space, power and the exclusion of disabled people. *Disability & Society, 13*, 343–356. doi:10.1080/09687599826678

Klein, S. D., & Schive, K. (2001). *You will dream new dreams: Inspiring personal stories by parents of children with disabilities.* New York, NY: Kensington.

Knestricht, T., & Kuchey, D. (2009). Welcome to Holland: Characteristics of resilient families raising children with severe disabilities. *Journal of Family Studies, 15*, 227–244. doi:10.5172/jfs.15.3.227

Kober, R., & Eggleton, I. R. C. (2005). The effect of different types of employment on quality of life. *Journal of Intellectual Disability Research, 49*, 756–760. doi:10.1111/j.1365-2788.2005.00746.x

Kogan, M. D., Strickland, B. B., & Newacheck, P. W. (2009). Building systems of care: Findings from the National Survey of Children with Special Care Needs. *Pediatrics, 124*, S333–S336. doi:10.1542/peds.2009-1255B

Kramer, J. (2009). I am not my brother's keeper. In D. Meyer (Ed.), *Thicker than water: Essays by adult siblings of people with disabilities* (pp. 20–26). Bethesda, MD: Woodbine House.

Krauss, M. W., & Seltzer, M. M. (1993). Current well-being and future plans of older caregiving mothers. *The Irish Journal of Psychology, 14*(1), 48–63. Retrieved from http://direct.bl.uk/bld/PlaceOrder.do?UIN=006535483&ETOC=EN&from= searchengine doi:10.1080/03033910.1993.10557914

Krauss, M. W., Seltzer, M. M., Gordon, R., & Friedman, D. H. (1996). Binding ties: The roles of adult siblings of persons with mental retardation. *Mental Retardation, 34*, 83–93. Retrieved from http://psycnet.apa.org/psycinfo/1997-38694-002

Lake, J. F., & Billingsley, B. S. (2000). An analysis of factors that contribute to parent–school conflict in special education. *Remedial and Special Education, 21*, 240–251. doi:10.1177/074193250002100407

Lane, H. (1976). *The wild boy of Aveyron.* Cambridge, MA: Harvard.

Lane, H. (1995). Constructions of deafness. *Disability & Society, 10*, 171–190. doi:10.1080/09687599550023633

Lasky, B., & Karge, B. D. (2011). Involvement of language minority parents of children with disabilities in their child's school achievement. *Multicultural Education, 18*, 29–34.

Lau, C., Hurst, N. M., Smith, E. O., & Schanler, R. J. (2007). Ethnic/racial diversity, maternal stress, lactation and very low birthweight infants. *Journal of Perinatology, 27*, 399–408. doi:10.1038/sj.jp.7211770

Lavee, Y., McCubbin, H. I., & Patterson, J. M. (1985). The double ABCX model of family stress and adaptation: An empirical test by analysis of structural equations with latent variables. *Journal of Marriage and the Family, 47*, 811–825. doi:10.2307/352326

Law, M., Hanna, S., King, G., Hurley, P., King, S., Kertoy, M., & Rosenbaum, P. (2003). Factors affecting family-centred service delivery for children with disabilities. *Child: Care, Health and Development, 29*, 357–366. doi:10.1046/j.1365-2214.2003.00351.x

Laws, G., & Milward, L. (2001). Predicting parents' satisfaction with the education of their child with Down's syndrome. *Educational Research, 43*, 209–226. doi:10.1080/0013188011005117 3

Lawson, H., Parker, M., & Sikes, P. (2006). Seeking stories: Reflections on a narrative approach to researching understandings of inclusion. *European Journal of Special Needs Education, 21*, 55–68. doi:10.1080/08856250500491823

Layous, K., Chancellor, J., Lyubomirsky, S., Wang, L., & Doraiswamy, P. M. (2011). Delivering happiness: Translating positive psychology intervention research for treating major and minor depressive disorders. *The Journal of Alternative and Complementary Medicine, 17*, 675–683. doi:10.1089/acm.2011.0139

Lazarus, R. S., & Folkman, S. (1984). *Stress, appraisal, and coping.* New York, NY: Springer.

Lecavalier, L., Leone, S., & Wiltz, J. (2006). The impact of behaviour problems on caregiver stress in young people with autism spectrum disorders. *Journal of Intellectual Disability Research, 50,* 172–183. doi:10.1111/j.1365-2788.2005.00732.x

Leigh, I. W., Powers, L., Vash, C., & Nettles, R. (2004). Survey of psychological services to clients with disabilities: The need for awareness. *Rehabilitation Psychology, 49,* 48–54. doi:10.1037/0090-5550.49.1.48

Leiter, V., & Krauss, M. W. (2004). Claims, barriers, and satisfaction: Parents' requests for additional special education services. *Journal of Disability Policy Studies, 15,* 135–146. doi:10.1177/10442073040150030201

Leiter, V., Krauss, M. W., Anderson, B., & Wells, N. (2004). The consequences of caring: Effects of mothering a child with special needs. *Journal of Family Issues, 25,* 379–403. doi:10.1177/0192513X03257415

Lenhard, W., Breitenbach, E., Ebert, H., Schindelhauer-Deutscher, H. J., & Henn, W. (2005). Psychological benefit of diagnostic certainty for mothers of children with disabilities. *American Journal of Medical Genetics, 133A,* 170–175. doi:10.1002/ajmg.a.30571

Lepore, S. J., Silver, R. C., Wortman, C. B., & Wayment, H. A. (1996). Social constraints, intrusive thoughts, and depressive symptoms among bereaved mothers. *Journal of Personality and Social Psychology, 70,* 271–282. doi:10.1037/0022-3514.70.2.271

Levy-Wasser, N., & Katz, S. (2004). The relationship between attachment style, birth order, and adjustment in children who grow up with a sibling with mental retardation. *British Journal of Developmental Disabilities, 50,* 89–98. doi:10.1179/096979504799103921

Lewis, S., Kagan, C., Heaton, P., & Cranshaw, M. (1999). Economic and psychological benefits from employment: The experiences and perspectives of mothers of disabled children. *Disability & Society, 14,* 561–575. doi:10.1080/09687599926127

Lewit, E. M., & Baker, L. S. (1996). Children in special education. *The Future of Children, 6,* 139–151. doi:10.2307/1602498

Linley, P. A., & Joseph, S. (2004). Positive change following trauma and adversity: A review. *Journal of Traumatic Stress, 17,* 11–21. doi:10.1023/B:JOTS.0000014671.27856.7e

Loevinger, J. (1985). Revision of the sentence completion test for ego development. *Journal of Personality and Social Psychology, 48,* 420–427. doi:10.1037/0022-3514.48.2.420

Lombardo, P. A. (2008). *Three generations, no imbeciles: Eugenics, the Supreme Court, and Buck v. Bell.* Baltimore, MD: Johns Hopkins.

Lord, B., Ungerer, J., & Wastell, C. (2008). Implications of resolving the diagnosis of PKU for parents and children. *Journal of Pediatric Psychology, 33,* 855–866. doi:10.1093/jpepsy/jsn020

Ly, T. M., & Hodapp, R. M. (2005). Children with Prader-Willi syndrome vs. Williams syndrome: Indirect effects on parents during a jigsaw puzzle task. *Jour-*

nal of Intellectual Disability Research, 49, 929–939. doi:10.1111/j.1365-2788. 2005.00782.x

Lyubomirsky, S., Sheldon, K. M., & Schkade, D. (2005). Pursuing happiness: The architecture of sustainable change. *Review of General Psychology, 9*, 111–131. doi:10.1037/1089-2680.9.2.111

MacDonald, H., & Callery, P. (2004). Different meanings of respite: A study of parents, nurses, and social workers caring for children with complex needs. *Child: Care, Health and Development, 30*, 279–288. doi:10.1111/j.1365-2214. 2004.00392.x

MacFarlane, J. R., & Kanaya, T. (2009). What does it mean to be autistic? Inter-state variation in education criteria for autism services. *Journal of Child and Family Studies, 18*, 662–669. doi:10.1007/s10826-009-9268-8

MacMullin, J. A., Viecili, M. A., Cappadocia, M. C., & Weiss, J. A. (2010). Brief report: Parent empowerment and mental health: Understanding parent perceptions of the educational experience. *Journal on Developmental Disabilities, 16*, 68–71. Retrieved from http://www.oadd.org/Published_Issues_142.html

Madriaga, M. (2010). "I avoid pubs and the student union like the plague": Students with Asperger syndrome and their negotiation of university spaces. *Children's Geographies, 8*, 39–50. doi:10.1080/14733280903500166

Magaña, S., Parish, S. L., Rose, R. A., Timberlake, M., & Swaine, J. G. (2012). Racial and ethnic disparities in quality of health care among children with autism and other developmental disabilities. *Intellectual and Developmental Disabilities, 50*, 287–299. doi:10.1352/1934-9556-50.4.287

Mandell, D. S., Listerud, J., Levy, S. E., & Pinto-Martin, J. A. (2002). Race differences in the age of diagnosis of Medicaid-eligible children with autism. *Journal of the American Academy of Child & Adolescent Psychiatry, 41*, 1447–1453. doi:10.1097/00004583-200212000-00016

Mandell, D. S., & Novak, M. (2005). The role of culture in families' treatment decisions for children with autism spectrum disorders. *Mental Retardation and Developmental Disabilities Research Reviews, 11*, 110–115. doi:10.1002/mrdd.20061

Mandell, D. S., Novak, M. M., & Zubritsky, C. D. (2005). Factors associated with age of diagnosis among children with autism spectrum disorders. *Pediatrics, 116*, 1480–1486. doi:10.1542/peds.2005-0185

Mandell, D. S., & Salzer, M. S. (2007). Who joins support groups among parents of children with autism? *Autism, 11*, 111–122. doi:10.1177/1362361307077506

Mandell, D. S., Wiggins, L. D., Carpenter, L. A., Daniels, J., DiGuiseppi, C., Durkin, M. S., . . . Kirby, R. S. (2009). Racial/ethnic disparities in the identification of children with autism spectrum disorders. *American Journal of Public Health, 99*, 493–498. doi:10.2105/AJPH.2007.131243

Mandlawitz, M. R. (2002). The impact of the legal system on educational programming for young children with autism spectrum disorder. *Journal of Autism and Developmental Disorders, 32*, 495–508. doi:10.1023/A:1020502324718

Maner, J. K., DeWall, C. N., Baumeister, R. F., & Schaller, M. (2007). Does social exclusion motivate interpersonal reconnection? Resolving the "porcupine problem." *Journal of Personality and Social Psychology, 92,* 42–55. doi:10.1037/0022-3514.92.1.42

Mangione-Smith, R., McGlynn, E. A., Elliott, M. N., Krogstad, P., & Brook, R. H. (1999). The relationship between perceived parental expectations and pediatrician antimicrobial prescribing behavior. *Pediatrics, 103,* 711–718. doi:10.1542/peds.103.4.711

Manuel, J., Naughton, M. J., Balkrishnan, R., Smith, B. P., & Koman, L. A. (2003). Stress and adaptation in mothers of children with cerebral palsy. *Journal of Pediatric Psychology, 28,* 197–201. doi:10.1093/jpepsy/jsg007

Marcenko, M. O., & Meyers, J. C. (1991). Mothers of children with developmental disabilities: Who shares the burden? *Family Relations, 40,* 186–190. doi:10.2307/585481

Marks, S. U., Matson, A., & Barraza, L. (2005). The impact of siblings with disabilities on their brothers and sisters pursuing a career in special education. *Research and Practice for Persons with Severe Disabilities, 30,* 205–218. doi:10.2511/rpsd.30.4.205

Marlow, N., Wolke, D., Bracewell, M. A., & Samara, M. (2005). Neurologic and developmental disability at six years of age after extremely preterm birth. *The New England Journal of Medicine, 352,* 9–19. doi:10.1056/NEJMoa041367

Martin, E. W., Martin, R., & Terman, D. L. (1996). The legislative and litigation history of special education. *The Future of Children, 6,* 25–39. doi:10.2307/1602492

Maynard, D. W. (2004). On predicating a diagnosis as an attribute of a person. *Discourse Studies, 6,* 53–76. doi:10.1177/1461445604039439

McAdams, D. P. (2001). The psychology of life stories. *Review of General Psychology, 5,* 100–122. doi:10.1037/1089-2680.5.2.100

McAdams, D. P. (2006). The redemptive self: Generativity and the stories Americans live by. *Research in Human Development, 3,* 81–100. doi:10.1080/15427609.2006.9683363

McAdams, D. P. (2008). Personal narratives and the life story. In O. John, R. Robins, & L. A. Pervin (Eds.), *Handbook of personality: Theory and research* (3rd ed., pp. 242–262). New York, NY: Guilford Press.

McAdams, D. P., & Bowman, P. J. (2001). Narrating life's turning points: Redemption and contamination. In D. P. McAdams, R. Josselson, & A. Lieblich (Eds.), *Turns in the road: Narrative studies of lives in transition* (pp. 3–34). Washington, DC: American Psychological Association. doi:10.1037/10410-001

McAdams, D. P., Diamond, A., de St. Aubin, E., & Mansfield, E. (1997). Stories of commitment: The psychosocial construction of generative lives. *Journal of Personality and Social Psychology, 72,* 678–694. doi:10.1037/0022-3514.72.3.678

McAdams, D. P., Hoffman, B. J., Mansfield, E. D., & Day, R. (1996). Themes of agency and communion in significant autobiographical scenes. *Journal of Personality, 64*, 339–377. doi:10.1111/j.1467-6494.1996.tb00514.x

McDermott-Perez, L. (2007). *Preemie parents: Recovering from baby's premature birth.* Westport, CT: Praeger.

McGowan, J. E., Alderdice, F. A., Holmes, V. A., & Johnston, L. (2011). Early childhood development of late-preterm infants: A systematic review. *Pediatrics, 127*, 1111–1124. doi:10.1542/peds.2010-2257

McHale, S. M., & Gamble, W. C. (1989). Sibling relationships of children with disabled and nondisabled brothers and sisters. *Developmental Psychology, 25*, 421–429. doi:10.1037/0012-1649.25.3.421

McHale, S. M., & Pawletko, T. M. (1992). Differential treatment of siblings in two family contexts. *Child Development, 63*, 68–81. doi:10.2307/1130902

McIntyre, L. L. (2008). Parent training for young children with developmental disabilities: Randomized controlled trial. *American Journal on Mental Retardation, 113*, 356–368. doi:10.1352/2008.113:356-368

McLanahan, S., & Adams, J. (1987). Parenthood and psychological well-being. *Annual Review of Sociology, 13*, 237–257. doi:10.1146/annurev.soc. 13.1.237

McManus, J. L., Feyes, K. J., & Saucier, D. A. (2011). Contact and knowledge as predictors of attitudes toward individuals with intellectual disabilities. *Journal of Social and Personal Relationships, 28*, 579–590. doi:10.1177/0265407510385494

McNulty, J. K. (2010). When positive processes hurt relationships. *Current Directions in Psychological Science, 19*, 167–171. doi:10.1177/0963721410370298

McPherson, M., Arango, P., Fox, H., Lauver, C., McManus, M., Newacheck, P. W., . . . Strickland, B. (1998). A new definition of children with special health care needs. *Pediatrics, 102*, 137–139. doi:10.1542/peds.102.1.137

Melnyk, B. M., Crean, H. F., Feinstein, N. F., & Fairbanks, E. (2008). Maternal anxiety and depression following discharge from the NICU: Explanatory effects of the COPE program. *Nursing Research, 57*, 383–394. doi:10.1097/NNR.0b013e3181906f59

Meyer, D. (2009). *Thicker than water: Essays by adult siblings of people with disabilities.* Bethesda, MD: Woodbine House.

Meyer, D. J. (1995). (Ed.). *Uncommon fathers: Reflections on raising a child with a disability.* Bethesda, MD: Woodbine House.

Michie, M., & Skinner, D. (2010). Narrating disability, narrating religious practice: Reconciliation and fragile X syndrome. *Intellectual and Developmental Disabilities, 48*, 99–111. doi:10.1352/1934-9556-48.2.99

Miles, M. S., & Funk, S. G. (1993). Parental stressor scale: Neonatal intensive care unit. *Nursing Research, 42*, 148–152. doi:10.1097/00006199-199305000-00005

Miles, M. S., Funk, S. G., & Kasper, M. A. (1991). The neonatal intensive care unit environment: Sources of stress for parents. *AACN Clinical Issues in Critical Care Nursing, 2*, 346–354. Retrieved from http://ukpmc.ac.uk/abstract/MED/2021521

Milner, P., & Kelly, B. (2009). Community participation and inclusion: People with disabilities defining their place. *Disability & Society, 24*, 47–62. doi:10.1080/09687590802535410

Milo, E. M. (1997). Maternal responses to the life and death of a child with a developmental disability: A story of hope. *Death Studies, 21*, 443–476. doi:10.1080/074811897201822

Milshtein, S., Yirmiya, N., Oppenheim, D., Koren-Karie, N., & Levi, S. (2010). Resolution of the diagnosis among parents of children with autism spectrum disorder: Associations with child and parent characteristics. *Journal of Autism and Developmental Disorders, 40*, 89–99. doi:10.1007/s10803-009-0837-x

Montes, G., & Halterman, J. S. (2007). Bullying among children with autism and the influence of comorbidity with ADHD: A population-based study. *Ambulatory Pediatrics, 7*, 253–257. doi:10.1016/j.ambp.2007.02.003

Montes, G., Halterman, J. S., & Magyar, C. I. (2009). Access to and satisfaction with school and community health services for US children with ASD. *Pediatrics, 124*, S407–S413. doi:10.1542/peds.2009-1255L

Morris, J. E., & Coley, R. L. (2004). Maternal, family, and work correlates of role strain in low-income mothers. *Journal of Family Psychology, 18*, 424–432. doi:10.1037/0893-3200.18.3.424

Muller-Nix, C., Forcada-Guex, M., Pierrehumbert, B., Jaunin, L., Borghini, A., & Ansermet, F. (2004). Prematurity, maternal stress and mother–child interactions. *Early Human Development, 79*, 145–158. doi:10.1016.j.earlhumdev.2004.05.002

Mulroy, S., Robertson, L., Aiberti, K., Leonard, H., & Bower, C. (2008). The impact of having a sibling with an intellectual disability: Parental perspectives in two disorders. *Journal of Intellectual Disability Research, 52*, 216–229. doi:10.1111/j.1365-2788.2007.01005.x

Murch, S. H., Anthony, A., Casson, D. H., Malik, M., Berelowitz, M., Dhilion, A. P., . . . Walker-Smith, J. A. (2004). Retraction of an interpretation. *The Lancet, 363*, 750. doi:10.1016/S0140-6736(04)15715-2

Myers, B. J., Mackintosh, V. H., & Goin-Kochel, R. P. (2009). "My greatest joy and my greatest heart ache": Parents' own words on how having a child in the autism spectrum has affected their lives and their families' lives. *Research in Autism Spectrum Disorders, 3*, 670–684. doi:10.1016/j.rasd.2009.01.004

Nassar, N., Dixon, G., Bourke, J., Bower, C., Glasson, E., de Klerk, N., & Leonard, H. (2009). Autism spectrum disorders in young children: Effects of changes in diagnostic practices. *International Journal of Epidemiology, 38*, 1245–1254. doi:10.1093/ije/dyp260

Neece, C. L., Blacher, J., & Baker, B. L. (2010). Impact on siblings of children with intellectual disability: The role of child behavior problems. *American Journal on Intellectual and Developmental Disabilities, 115*, 291–306. doi:10.1352/1944-7558-115.4.291

Neimeyer, R. A. (2000). Searching for the meaning of meaning: Grief therapy and the process of reconstruction. *Death Studies, 24,* 541–558. doi:10.1080/07481180050121480

Neugebauer, R. (1978). Treatment of the mentally ill in medieval and early modern England: A reappraisal. *Journal of the History of the Behavioral Sciences, 14,* 158–169. doi:10.1002/1520-6696(197804)14:2<158::AID-JHBS 2300140209>3.0.CO;2-C

Newacheck, P. W., Hughes, D. C., Hung, Y.-Y., Wong, S., & Stoddard, J. J. (2000). The unmet health needs of America's children. *Pediatrics, 105,* 989–997. doi:10.1542/peds.105.4.S1.989

Newacheck, P. W., Inkelas, M., & Kim, S. E. (2004). Health services use and health care expenditures for children with disabilities. *Pediatrics, 114,* 79–85. doi:10.1542/peds.114.1.79

Newacheck, P. W., & Kim, S. E. (2005). A national profile of health care utilization and expenditures for children with special health care needs. *Archives of Pediatrics & Adolescent Medicine, 159,* 10–17. doi:10.1001/archpedi.159.1.10

Newcomb, A. F., Bukowski, W. M., & Pattee, L. (1993). Children's peer relations: A meta-analytic review of popular, rejected, neglected, controversial, and average sociometric status. *Psychological Bulletin, 113,* 99–128. doi:10.1037/0033-2909.113.1.99

Newschaffer, C. J., Croen, L. A., Daniels, J., Giarelli, E., Grether, J. K., Levy, S. E., . . . Windham, G. C. (2007). The epidemiology of autism spectrum disorders. *Annual Review of Public Health, 28,* 235–258. doi:10.1146/annurev.publhealth.28.021406.144007

Niccols, A., & Mohamed, S. (2000). Parent training in groups: Pilot study with parents of infants with developmental delay. *Journal of Early Intervention, 23,* 133–143. doi:10.1177/105381510002300207

Nixon, C. D., & Singer, G. H. S. (1993). Group cognitive-behavioral treatment for excessive parental self-blame and guilt. *American Journal on Mental Retardation, 97,* 665–672. Retrieved from http://direct.bl.uk/bld/PlaceOrder.do?UIN=0065 08716&ETOC=EN&from=searchengine

Nolan, K. W., Orlando, M., & Liptak, G. S. (2007). Care coordination services for children with special health care needs: Are we family-centered yet? *Families, Systems, & Health, 25,* 293–306. doi:10.1037/1091-7527.25.3.293

Nolen-Hoeksema, S., McBride, A., & Larson, J. (1997). Rumination and psychological distress among bereaved partners. *Journal of Personality and Social Psychology, 72,* 855–862. doi:10.1037/0022-3514.72.4.855

Noyes, J. (2000). Enabling young "ventilator-dependent" people to express their views and experiences of their care in hospital. *Journal of Advanced Nursing, 31,* 1206–1215. doi:10.1046/j.1365-2648.2000.01376.x

Obeidat, H. M., Bond, E. A., & Callister, L. C. (2009). The parental experience of having an infant in the newborn intensive care unit. *Journal of Perinatal Education, 18,* 23–29. doi:10.1624/105812409X461199

O'Connor, U. (2008). Meeting in the middle? A study of parent–professional partnerships. *European Journal of Special Needs Education, 23,* 253–268. doi:10.1080/08856250802130434

Odom, S. L., Zercher, C., Li, S., Marquart, J. M., Sandall, S., & Brown, W. H. (2006). Social acceptance and rejection of preschool children with disabilities: A mixed-method analysis. *Journal of Educational Psychology, 98,* 807–823. doi:10.1037/0022-0663.98.4.807

Olivos, E. M., Gallagher, R. J., & Aguilar, J. (2010). Fostering collaboration with culturally and linguistically diverse families of children with moderate to severe disabilities. *Journal of Educational & Psychological Consultation, 20,* 28–40. doi:10.1080/10474410903535372

Olkin, R. (2002). Can you hold the door open for me? Including disability in diversity. *Cultural Diversity and Ethnic Minority Psychology, 8,* 130–137. doi:10.1037/1099-9809.8.2.130

Olkin, R., & Pledger, C. (2003). Can disability studies and psychology join hands? *American Psychologist, 58,* 296–304. doi:10.1037/0003-066X.58.4.296

Ollendick, T. H., Weist, M. D., Borden, M. C., & Greene, R. W. (1992). Sociometric status and academic, behavioral, and psychological adjustment: A five-year longitudinal study. *Journal of Consulting and Clinical Psychology, 60,* 80–87. doi:10.1037/0022-006X.60.1.80

Olshansky, S. (1962). Chronic sorrow: A response to having a mentally defective child. *Social Casework, 43,* 191–193.

O'Mahar, K., Holmbeck, G. N., Jandasek, B., & Zukerman, J. (2010). A camp-based intervention targeting independence among individuals with spina bifida. *Journal of Pediatric Psychology, 35,* 848–856. doi:10.1093/jpepsy/jsp125

Oppenheim, D., Koren-Karie, N., Dolev, S., & Yirmiya, N. (2009). Maternal insightfulness and resolution of the diagnosis are associated with secure attachment in preschoolers with autism spectrum disorders. *Child Development, 80,* 519–527. doi:10.1111/j.1467-8624.2009.01276.x

Orsmond, G. I., & Seltzer, M. M. (2007). Siblings of individuals with autism or Down syndrome: Effects on adult lives. *Journal of Intellectual Disability Research, 51,* 682–696. doi:10.1111/j.1365-2788.2007.00954.x

Orsmond, G. I., & Seltzer, M. M. (2009). Adolescent siblings of individuals with an autism spectrum disorder: Testing a diathesis–stress model of sibling well-being. *Journal of Autism and Developmental Disorders, 39,* 1053–1065. doi:10.1007/s10803-009-0722-7

Orsmond, G. I., Seltzer, M. M., Greenberg, J. S., & Krauss, M. W. (2006). Mother–child relationship quality among adolescents and adults with autism. *American Journal on Mental Retardation, 111,* 121–137. doi:10.1352/0895-8017(2006)111[121:MRQAAA]2.0.CO;2

Ouellette-Kuntz, H., Burge, P., Brown, H. K., & Arsenault, E. (2010). Public attitudes toward individuals with intellectual disabilities as measured by the concept of social distance. *Journal of Applied Research in Intellectual Disabilities, 23*, 132–142. doi:10.1111/j.1468-3148.2009.00514.x

Ozonoff, S., Young, G. S., Steinfeld, M. B., Hill, M. M., Cook, I., Hutman, T., . . . Sigman, M. (2009). How early do parent concerns predict later autism diagnosis? *Journal of Developmental and Behavioral Pediatrics, 30*, 367–375. doi:10.1097/DBP.0b013e3181ba0fcf

Paczkowski, E., & Baker, B. L. (2008). Parenting children with developmental delays: The role of positive beliefs. *Journal of Mental Health Research in Intellectual Disabilities, 1*(3), 156–175. doi:10.1080/19315860801988392

Pain, H. (1999). Coping with a child with disabilities from the parents' perspective: The function of information. *Child: Care, Health and Development, 25*, 299–313. doi:10.1046/j.1365-2214.1999.00132.x

Palmer, D. S., Fuller, K., Arora, T., & Nelson, M. (2001). Taking sides: Parent views on inclusion for their children with severe disabilities. *Exceptional Children, 67*, 467–484. Retrieved from http://cec.metapress.com/content/u72256mx52p7/?p=302c478058794ac7847240ea031fccae&pi=43

Parish, S., Magaña, S., Rose, R., Timberlake, M., & Swaine, J. G. (2012). Health care of Latino children with autism and other developmental disabilities: Quality of provider interaction mediates utilization. *American Journal on Intellectual and Developmental Disabilities, 117*, 304–315. doi:10.1352/1944-7558-117.4.304

Parish, S. L. (2006). Juggling and struggling: A preliminary work-life study of mothers with adolescents who have developmental disabilities. *Mental Retardation, 44*, 393–404. doi:10.1352/0047-6765(2006)44[393:JASAPW]2.0.CO;2

Parish, S. L., & Cloud, J. M. (2006). Financial well-being of young children with disabilities and their families. *Social Work, 51*, 223–232. doi:10.1093/sw/51.3.223

Parish, S. L., Rose, R. A., & Swaine, J. G. (2010). Financial well-being of US parents caring for coresident children and adults with developmental disabilities: An age cohort analysis. *Journal of Intellectual and Developmental Disability, 35*, 235–243. doi:10.3109/13668250.2010.519331

Parish, S. L., Seltzer, M. M., Greenberg, J. S., & Floyd, F. (2004). Economic implications of caregiving at midlife: Comparing parents with and without children who have developmental disabilities. *Mental Retardation, 42*, 413–426. doi:10.1352/0047-6765(2004)42<413:EIOCAM>2.0.CO;2

Park, C. L. (2010). Making sense of the meaning literature: An integrative review of meaning making and its effects on adjustment to stressful life events. *Psychological Bulletin, 136*, 257–301. doi:10.1037/a0018301

Park, N., Peterson, C., & Seligman, M. P. (2006). Character strengths in fifty-four nations and the fifty US states. *The Journal of Positive Psychology, 1*, 118–129. doi:10.1080/17439760600619567

Parke, R. D., McDowell, D. J., Cladis, M., & Leidy, M. S. (2006). Family and peer relationships: The role of emotion regulatory processes. In D. K. Snyder, J. Simpson, & J. N. Hughes (Eds.), *Emotion regulation in couples and families:*

Pathways to dysfunction and health (pp. 143–162). Washington, DC: American Psychological Association. doi:10.1037/11468-007

Parsons, T. (1951). *The social system*. Glencoe, IL: Free Press.

Parsons, T. (1975). The sick role and the role of physician reconsidered. *Health and Society, 53,* 257–278. Retrieved from http://www.jstor.org/discover/10.2307/33 49493?uid=3739736&uid=2&uid=4&uid=3739256&sid=47698945969727

Patja, K., Iivanainen, M., Vesala, H., Oksanen, H., & Ruoppila, I. (2000). Life expectancy of people with intellectual disability: A 35-year follow-up study. *Journal of Intellectual Disability Research, 44,* 591–599. doi:10.1046/j.1365-2788.2000.00280.x

Pennebaker, J. W., Booth, M. J., & Francis, M. E. (2007). *Linguistic inquiry and word count.* Austin, TX: LIWC.net.

Pennebaker, J. W., & Francis, M. E. (1996). Cognitive, emotional, and language processes in disclosure. *Cognition and Emotion, 10,* 601–626. doi:10.1080/026999396380079

Pennebaker, J. W., Mayne, T. J., & Francis, M. E. (1997). Linguistic predictors of adaptive bereavement. *Journal of Personality and Social Psychology, 72,* 863–871. doi:10.1037/0022-3514.72.4.863

Pennebaker, J. W., Mehl, M. R., & Niederhoffer, K. G. (2003). Psychological aspects of natural language use: Our words, our selves. *Annual Review of Psychology, 54,* 547–577. doi:10.1146/annurev.psych.54.101601.145041

Perakyla, A. (1997). Conversation analysis: A new model of research in doctor–patient communication. *Journal of the Royal Society of Medicine, 90,* 205–208. Retrieved from http://jrsm.rsmjournals.com/content/90/4.toc

Perry, A., Harris, K., & Minnes, P. (2004). Family environments and family harmony: An exploration across severity, age, and type of DD. *Journal on Developmental Disabilities, 11,* 17–29. Retrieved from http://www.oadd.org/Published_Issues_142.html

Petalas, M. A., Hastings, R. P., Nash, S., Lloyd, T., & Dowey, A. (2009). Emotional and behavioural adjustment in siblings of children with intellectual disability with and without autism. *Autism, 13,* 471–483. doi:10.1177/1362361309335721

Peterson, C., Park, N., Pole, N., D'Andrea, W., & Seligman, M. E. P. (2008). Strengths of character and posttraumatic growth. *Journal of Traumatic Stress, 21,* 214–217. doi:10.1002/jts.20332

Peterson, C., & Vaidya, R. S. (2003). Optimism as vice and virtue. In E. C. Chang & L. J. Sanna (Eds.), *Virtue, vice, and personality: The complexity of behavior* (pp. 23–37). Washington, DC: American Psychological Association. doi:10.1037/10614-002

Phelps, L. A., & Hanley-Maxwell, C. (1997). School-to-work transitions for youth with disabilities: A review of outcomes and practices. *Review of Educational Research, 67,* 197–226. doi:10.2307/1170626

Pierrehumbert, B., Nicole, A., Muller-Nix, C., Forcada-Guex, M., & Ansermet, F. (2003). Parental post-traumatic reactions after premature birth: Implications for sleeping and eating problems in the infant. *Archives of Disease in Childhood. Fetal and Neonatal Edition, 88*, F400–F404. doi:10.1136/fn.88.5.F400

Pisterman, S., Firestone, P., McGrath, P., Goodman, J. T., Webster, I., Mallory, R., & Goffin, B. (1992). The effects of parenting training on parenting stress and sense of competence. *Canadian Journal of Behavioural Science/ Revue canadienne des sciences du comportement, 24*, 41–58. doi:10.1037/ h0078699

Pisterman, S., McGrath, P., Firestone, P., Goodman, J. T., Webster, I., & Mallory, R. (1989). Outcome of parent-mediated treatment of preschoolers with attention deficit disorder with hyperactivity. *Journal of Consulting and Clinical Psychology, 57*, 628–635. doi:10.1037/0022-006X.57.5.628

Plant, K. M., & Sanders, M. R. (2007). Predictors of care-giver stress in families of preschool-aged children with developmental disabilities. *Journal of Intellectual Disability Research, 51*, 109–124. doi:10.1111/j.1365-2788.2006.00829.x

Podell, D. M., & Soodak, L. C. (1993). Teacher efficacy and bias in special education referrals. *The Journal of Educational Research, 86*, 247–253. doi:10.1080/00220 671.1993.9941836

Praisner, C. L. (2003). Attitudes of elementary school principals toward the inclusion of students with disabilities. *Exceptional Children, 69*, 135–145. Retrieved from http://cec.metapress.com/content/l40l57113121/?p=ce1317719b9745dc9 66a2f11b74acde9&pi=37

Pruchno, R. A. (2003). Enmeshed lives: Adult children with developmental disabilities and their aging mothers. *Psychology and Aging, 18*, 851–857. doi:10.1037/0882-7974.18.4.851

Quinn, M., Carr, A., Carroll, L., & O'Sullivan, D. (2007). Parents plus programme I: Evaluation of its effectiveness for pre-school children with developmental disabilities and behavioural problems. *Journal of Applied Research in Intellectual Disabilities, 20*, 345–359. doi:10.1111/j.1468-3148.2006.00352.x

Quinn, M. M., Rutherford, R. B., Leone, P. E., Osher, D. M., & Poirer, J. M. (2005). Youth with disabilities in juvenile corrections: A national survey. *Exceptional Children, 71*(3), 339–345. Retrieved from http://www.arturohernandez.org/ disability-best_corrections_survey.pdf

Quinnell, F. A., & Hynan, M. T. (1999). Convergent and discriminant validity of the perinatal PTSD questionnaire (PPQ): A preliminary study. *Journal of Traumatic Stress, 12*, 193–199. doi:10.1023/A:1024714903950

Rademaker, A. R., van Zuiden, M., Vermetten, E., & Geuze, E. (2011). Type D personality and the development of PTSD symptoms: A prospective study. *Journal of Abnormal Psychology, 120*, 299–307. doi:10.1037/a0021806

Reder, E. A., & Serwint, J. R. (2009). Until the last breath: Exploring the concept of hope for parents and health care professionals during a child's serious illness. *Archives of Pediatrics & Adolescent Medicine, 163*, 653–657. doi:10.1001/ archpediatrics.2009.87

Reed, G. L., & Enright, R. D. (2006). The effects of forgiveness therapy on depression, anxiety, and posttraumatic stress for women after spousal emotional abuse. *Journal of Consulting and Clinical Psychology, 74*, 920–929. doi:10.1037/0022-006X.74.5.920

Rehabilitation Act of 1973, Section 504, 29 U.S.C. Sec. 974 Retrieved from http://www.dol.gov/oasam/regs/statutes/sec504.htm#.UO2XW44qYVw

Rehm, R. S., & Bradley, J. F. (2005). Normalization in families raising a child who is medically fragile/technology dependent and developmentally delayed. *Qualitative Health Research, 15*, 807–820. doi:10.1177/1049732305276754

Reilly, D., Huws, J., Hastings, R., & Vaughan, F. (2010). Life and death of a child with Down syndrome and a congenital heart condition: Experiences of six couples. *Intellectual and Developmental Disabilities, 48*, 403–416. doi:10.1352/1934-9556-48.6.403

Reilly, D. E., Hastings, R. P., Vaughan, F. L., & Huws, J. C. (2008). Parental bereavement and the loss of a child with intellectual disabilities: A review of the literature. *Intellectual and Developmental Disabilities, 46*, 27–43. doi:10.1352/0047-6765(2008)46[27:PBATLO]2.0.CO;2

Reilly, D. E., Huws, J. C., Hastings, R. P., & Vaughan, F. L. (2008). "When your child dies you don't belong in that world any more"—Experiences of mothers whose child with an intellectual disability has died. *Journal of Applied Research in Intellectual Disabilities, 21*, 546–560. doi:10.1111/j.1468-3148.2008.00427.x

Rentinck, I., Ketelaar, M., Jongmans, M., Lindeman, E., & Gorter, J. W. (2009). Parental reactions following the diagnosis of cerebral palsy in their young child. *Journal of Pediatric Psychology, 34*, 671–676. doi:10.1093/jpepsy/jsn103

Rentinck, I. C. M., Ketelaar, M., Schuengel, C., Stolk, J., Lindeman, E., Jongmans, M., & Gorter, J. W. (2010). Short-term changes in parents' resolution regarding their young child's diagnosis of cerebral palsy. *Child: Care, Health and Development, 36*, 703–708. doi:10.1111/j.1365-2214.2010.01077.x

Resch, J. A., Mireles, G., Benz, M. R., Grenwelge, C., Peterson, R., & Zhang, D. (2010). Giving parents a voice: A qualitative study of the challenges experienced by parents of children with disabilities. *Rehabilitation Psychology, 55*, 139–150. doi:10.1037/a0019473

Retzlaff, R. (2007). Families of children with Rett syndrome: Stories of coherence and resilience. *Families, Systems, & Health, 25*, 246–262. doi:10.1037/1091-7527.25.3.246

Risdal, D., & Singer, G. H. S. (2004). Marital adjustment in parents of children with disabilities: A historical review and meta-analysis. *Research and Practice for Persons with Severe Disabilities, 29*, 95–103. doi:10.2511/rpsd.29.2.95

Rivers, J. W., & Stoneman, Z. (2003). Sibling relationships when a child has autism: Marital stress and support coping. *Journal of Autism and Developmental Disorders, 33*, 383–394. doi:10.1023/A:1025006727395

Roberts, C., Mazzucchelli, T., Studman, L., & Sanders, M. R. (2006). Behavioral family intervention for children with developmental disabilities and behavioral problems. *Journal of Clinical Child and Adolescent Psychology, 35*, 180–193. doi:10.1207/s15374424jccp3502_2

Robinson-Whelen, S., Tada, Y., MacCallum, R. C., McGuire, L., & Kiecolt-Glaser, J. K. (2001). Long-term caregiving: What happens when it ends? *Journal of Abnormal Psychology, 110*, 573–584. doi:10.1037/0021-843X.110.4.573

Rogers, C. H., Floyd, F. J., Seltzer, M. M., Greenberg, J., & Hong, J. (2008). Long-term effects of the death of a child on parents' adjustment in midlife. *Journal of Family Psychology, 22*, 203–211. doi:10.1037/0893-3200.22.2.203

Roll-Pettersson, L. (2001). Parents talk about how it feels to have a child with a cognitive disability. *European Journal of Special Needs Education, 16*, 1–14. doi:10.1080/08856250150501761

Rose, B. M., & Holmbeck, G. N. (2007). Attention and executive functions in adolescents with spina bifida. *Journal of Pediatric Psychology, 32*, 983–994. doi:10.1093/jpepsy/jsm042 doi:10.1093/jpepsy/jsm042

Rossiter, L., & Sharpe, D. (2001). The siblings of individuals with mental retardation: A quantitative integration of the literature. *Journal of Child and Family Studies, 10*, 65–84. doi:10.1023/A:1016629500708

Rueda, R., Monzo, L., Shapiro, J., Gomez, J., & Blacher, J. (2005). Latina mothers of young adults with developmental disabilities. *Exceptional Children, 71*, 401–414.

Runswick-Cole, K. (2010). Living with dying and disablism: Death and disabled children. *Disability & Society, 25*, 813–826. doi:10.1080/09687599.2010.520895

Russell, F. (2003). The expectations of parents of disabled children. *British Journal of Special Education, 30*, 144–149. doi:10.1111/1467-8527.00300

Ryan, S., & Cole, K. R. (2009). From advocate to activist? Mapping the experiences of mothers of children on the autism spectrum. *Journal of Applied Research in Intellectual Disabilities, 22*, 43–53. doi:10.1111/j.1468-3148.2008.00438.x

Salt, J., Shemilt, J., Sellars, V., Boyd, S., Coulson, T., & McCool, S. (2002). The Scottish Centre for Autism preschool treatment programme II: The results of a controlled treatment outcome study. *Autism, 6*, 33–46. doi:10.1177/1362361302006001004

Sameroff, A. (2009). The transactional model. In A. Sameroff (Ed.), *The transactional model of development: How children and contexts shape each other* (pp. 3–21). Washington, DC: American Psychological Association. doi:10.1037/11877-001

Samios, C. M., Pakenham, K. I., & Sofronoff, K. (2012). Sense making and benefit finding in couples who have a child with Asperger syndrome: An application of the actor–partner interdependence model. *Autism, 16*, 275–292. doi:10.1177/1362361311418691

Sanford, C., Newman, L., Wagner, M., Cameto, R., Knokey, A.-M., & Shaver, D. (2011). *The post–high school outcomes of young adults with disabilities up to 6 years after high school. Key findings from the National Longitudinal Transition Study-2*

(*NLTS2*). Menlo Park, CA: SRI International. Retrieved from http://policy web.sri.com/cehs/publications/publications.jsp

Santelli, B., Turnbull, A. P., Marquis, J., & Lerner, E. (1997). Parent-to-parent programs: A resource for parents and professionals. *Journal of Early Intervention, 21*, 73–83. doi:10.1177/105381519702100108

Santelli, B., Turnbull, A. P., Marquis, J. G., & Lerner, E. P. (1995). Parent to parent programs: A unique form of mutual support. *Infants and Young Children, 8*, 48–57. doi:10.1097/00001163-199510000-00007

Scallan, S., Senior, J., & Reilly, C. (2011). Williams syndrome: Daily challenges and positive impact on the family. *Journal of Applied Research in Intellectual Disabilities, 24*, 181–188. doi:10.1111/j.1468-3148.2010.00575.x

Schalock, R. L. (2000). Three decades of quality of life. *Focus on Autism and Other Developmental Disabilities, 15*, 116–127. doi:10.1177/108835760001500207

Schalock, R. L. (2004). The concept of quality of life: What we know and do not know. *Journal of Intellectual Disability Research, 48*, 203–216. doi:10.1111/j.1365-2788.2003.00558.x

Schalock, R. L., Luckasson, R. A., & Shogren, K. A. (2007). The renaming of *Mental Retardation*: Understanding the change to the term *Intellectual Disability*. *Intellectual and Developmental Disabilities, 45*, 116–124. doi:10.1352/1934-9556(2007)45[116:TROMRU]2.0.CO;2

Schormans, A. F. (2004). Experiences following the deaths of disabled foster children: "We don't feel like 'foster' parents". *Omega, 49*, 347–369. doi:10.2190/PMPX-5JWW-7LAB-C9LE

Schuengel, C., Rentinck, I. C. M., Stolk, J., Voorman, J. M., Loots, G. M. P., Ketelaar, M., . . . Becher, J. G. (2009). Parents' reaction to the diagnosis of cerebral palsy: Associations between resolution, age and severity of disability. *Child: Care, Health and Development, 35*, 673–680. doi:10.1111/j.1365-2214.2009.00951.x

Scorgie, K., & Sobsey, D. (2000). Transformational outcomes associated with parenting children who have disabilities. *Mental Retardation, 38*, 195–206. doi:10.1352/0047-6765(2000)038<0195:TOAWPC>2.0.CO;2

Seligman, M. E. P., & Csikszentmihalyi, M. (2000). Positive psychology: An introduction. *American Psychologist, 55*, 5–14. doi:10.1037/0003-066X.55.1.5

Seligman, M. E. P., Rashid, T., & Parks, A. C. (2006). Positive psychotherapy. *American Psychologist, 61*, 774–788. doi:10.1037/0003-066X.61.8.774

Seligman, M. E. P., Steen, T. A., Park, N., & Peterson, C. (2005). Positive psychology progress: Empirical validation of interventions. *American Psychologist, 60*, 410–421. doi:10.1037/0003-066X.60.5.410

Seltzer, M. M., Greenberg, J. S., Floyd, F. J., & Hong, J. (2004). Accommodative coping and well-being of midlife parents of children with mental health problems or developmental disabilities. *American Journal of Orthopsychiatry, 74*, 187–195. doi:10.1037/0002-9432.74.2.187

Seltzer, M. M., Greenberg, J. S., & Krauss, M. W. (1995). A comparison of coping strategies of aging mothers of adults with mental illness or mental retardation. *Psychology and Aging, 10*, 64–75. doi:10.1037/0882-7974.10.1.64

Seltzer, M. M., Greenberg, J. S., Krauss, M. W., Gordon, R. M., & Judge, K. (1997). Siblings of adults with mental retardation or mental illness: Effects on lifestyle and psychological well-being. *Family Relations, 46*, 395–405. doi:10.2307/585099

Seltzer, M. M., Greenberg, J. S., Orsmond, G. I., & Lounds, J. (2005). Life course studies of siblings of individuals with developmental disabilities. *Mental Retardation, 43*, 354–359. Retrieved from http://www.waisman.wisc.edu/family/pubs/Autism/2005%20Life%20course%20study%20sibs%20of%20indv%20with%20dd.pdf

Seltzer, M. M., Krauss, M. W., Hong, J., & Orsmond, G. I. (2001). Continuity or discontinuity of family involvement following residential transitions of adults who have mental retardation. *Mental Retardation, 39*, 181–194. doi:10.1352/0047-6765(2001)039<0181:CODOFI>2.0.CO;2

Selye, H. (1976). *The stress of life.* New York, NY: McGraw-Hill.

Shattuck, P. T. (2006). The contribution of diagnostic substitution to the growing administrative prevalence of autism in US special education. *Pediatrics, 117*, 1028–1037. doi:10.1542/peds.2005-1516

Shattuck, P. T., Durkin, M., Maenner, M., Newschaffer, C., Mandell, D., Wiggins, L., . . . Cuniff, C. (2009). Timing of identification among children with an autism spectrum disorder: Findings from a population-based surveillance study. *Journal of the American Academy of Child & Adolescent Psychiatry, 48*, 474–483. doi:10.1097/CHI.0b013e31819b3848

Shattuck, P. T., & Grosse, S. D. (2007). Issues related to the diagnosis and treatment of autism spectrum disorders. *Mental Retardation and Developmental Disabilities Research Reviews, 13*, 129–135. doi:10.1002/mrdd.20143

Shattuck, P. T., Seltzer, M. M., Greenberg, J. S., Orsmond, G. I., Bolt, D., Kring, S., . . . Lord, C. (2007). Change in autistic symptoms and maladaptive behaviors in adolescents and adults with an autism spectrum disorder. *Journal of Autism and Developmental Disorders, 37*, 1735–1747. doi:10.1007/s10803-006-0307-7

Shaw, D. S., Gross, H. E., & Moilanen, K. L. (2009). Developmental transactions between boys' conduct problems and mothers' depressive symptoms. In A. Sameroff (Ed.), *The transactional model of development: How children and contexts shape each other* (pp. 77–96). Washington, DC: American Psychological Association. doi:10.1037/11877-005

Shearn, J., & Todd, S. (2000). Maternal employment and family responsibilities: The perspectives of mothers of children with intellectual disabilities. *Journal of Applied Research in Intellectual Disabilities, 13*, 109–131. doi:10.1046/j.1468-3148.2000.00021.x

Sheeran, T., Marvin, R. S., & Pianta, R. C. (1997). Mothers' resolution of their child's diagnosis and self-reported measures of parenting stress, marital relations, and social support. *Journal of Pediatric Psychology*, *22*, 197–212. doi:10.1093/jpepsy/22.2.197

Sheets, K. B., Best, R. G., Brasington, C. K., & Will, M. C. (2011). Balanced information about Down syndrome: What is essential? *American Journal of Medical Genetics*, *155A*, 1246–1257. doi:10.1002/ajmg.a.34018

Shelden, D. L., Angell, M. E., Stoner, J. B., & Roseland, B. D. (2010). School principals' influence on trust: Perspectives of mothers of children with disabilities. *The Journal of Educational Research*, *103*, 159–170. doi:10.1080/00220670903382921

Shilling, V., Edwards, V., Rogers, M., & Morris, C. (2012). The experience of disabled children as inpatients: A structured review and synthesis of qualitative studies reporting the views of children, parents, and professionals. *Child: Care, Health and Development*, *38*, 778–788. doi:10.1111/j.1365-2214.2012.01372.x

Shu, B.-C., & Lung, F.-W. (2005). The effect of support group on the mental health and quality of life for mothers with autistic children. *Journal of Intellectual Disability Research*, *49*, 47–53. doi:10.1111/j.1365-2788.2005.00661.x

Simmerman, S., Blacher, J., & Baker, B. L. (2001). Fathers' and mothers' perceptions of father involvement in families with young children with a disability. *Journal of Intellectual and Developmental Disability*, *26*, 325–338. doi:10.1080/13668250120087335

Simons, R. (1987). *After the tears: Parents talk about raising a child with a disability*. Denver, CO: The Children's Museum of Denver.

Sin, N. L., & Lyubomirsky, S. (2009). Enhancing well-being and alleviating depressive symptoms with positive psychology interventions: A practice-friendly meta-analysis. *Journal of Clinical Psychology*, *65*, 467–487. doi:10.1002/jclp.20593

Singer, G. H. S. (2002). Suggestions for a pragmatic program of research on families and disability. *The Journal of Special Education*, *36*, 150–156. doi:10.1177/00224669020360030501

Singer, G. H. S. (2006). Meta-analysis of comparative studies of depression in mothers of children with and without developmental disabilities. *American Journal on Mental Retardation*, *111*, 155–169. doi:10.1352/0895-8017(2006)111[155:MOCSOD]2.0.CO;2

Singer, G. H. S., Ethridge, B. L., & Aldana, S. I. (2007). Primary and secondary effects of parenting and stress management interventions for parents of children with developmental disabilities: A meta-analysis. *Mental Retardation and Developmental Disabilities Research Reviews*, *13*, 357–369. doi:10.1002/mrdd.20175

Singer, G. H. S., Marquis, J., Powers, L. K., Blanchard, L., Divenere, N., Santelli, B., . . . Sharp, M. (1999). A multi-site evaluation of parent to parent programs for parents of children with disabilities. *Journal of Early Intervention*, *22*, 217–229. doi:10.1177/105381519902200305

Siperstein, G. N., Glick, G. C., & Parker, R. C. (2009). Social inclusion of children with intellectual disabilities in a recreational setting. *Intellectual and Developmental Disabilities, 47,* 97–107. doi: http://dx.doi.org/10.1352/1934-9556-47.2.97

Skinner, D., Bailey, D. B., Jr., Correa, V., & Rodriguez, P. (1999). Narrating self and disability: Latino mothers' construction of identities vis-à-vis their child with special needs. *Exceptional Children, 65,* 481–495. Retrieved from http://www.cec.sped.org/content/NavigationMenu/Publications2/exceptionalchildren/

Skotko, B. G., Capone, G. T., & Kishnani, P. S. (2009). Postnatal diagnosis of Down syndrome: Synthesis of the evidence of how best to deliver the news. *Pediatrics, 124,* e751–e758. doi:10.1542/peds.2009-0480

Skotko, B. G., & Levine, S. P. (2006). What the other children are thinking: Brothers and sisters of persons with Down syndrome. *American Journal of Medical Genetics, 142C,* 180–186. doi:10.1002/ajmg.c.30101

Smith, L. E., Greenberg, J. S., Seltzer, M. M., & Hong, J. (2008). Symptoms and behavior problems of adolescents and adults with autism: Effects of mother–child relationship quality, warmth, and praise. *American Journal on Mental Retardation, 113,* 387–402. doi:10.1352/2008.113:387-402

Smith, T. B., Oliver, M. N. I., & Innocenti, M. S. (2001). Parenting stress in families of children with disabilities. *American Journal of Orthopsychiatry, 71,* 257–261. doi:10.1037/0002-9432.71.2.257

Sofronoff, K., Dark, E., & Stone, V. (2011). Social vulnerability and bullying in children with Asperger syndrome. *Autism, 15,* 355–372 doi:10.1177/1362361310365070

Solomon, M., Pistrang, N., & Barker, C. (2001). The benefits of mutual support groups for parents of children with disabilities. *American Journal of Community Psychology, 29,* 113–132. doi:10.1023/A:1005253514140

Soodak, L. C., & Erwin, E. J. (1995). Parents, professionals, and inclusive education: A call for collaboration. *Journal of Educational & Psychological Consultation, 6,* 257–276. doi:10.1207/s1532768xjepc0603_6

Soodak, L. C., & Podell, D. M. (1994). Teachers' thinking about difficult-to-teach students. *The Journal of Educational Research, 88,* 44–51. doi:10.1080/0022067 1.1994.9944833

Soodak, L. C., Podell, D. M., & Lehman, L. R. (1998). Teacher, student, and school attributes as predictors of teachers' responses to inclusion. *The Journal of Special Education, 31,* 480–497. doi:10.1177/002246699803100405

Soper, K. L. (Ed.). (2007). *Gifts: Mothers reflect on how children with Down syndrome enrich their lives.* Bethesda, MD: Woodbine House.

Spagnola, M., & Fiese, B. H. (2007). Family routines and rituals: A context for development in the lives of young children. *Infants & Young Children, 20,* 284–299. doi:10.1097/01.IYC.0000290352.32170.5a

Spann, S. J., Kohler, F. W., & Soenksen, D. (2003). Examining parents' involvement in and perceptions of special education services: An interview with families in a parent support group. *Focus on Autism and Other Developmental Disabilities, 18,* 228–237. doi:10.1177/10883576030180040401

Stainton, T. (2001). Medieval charitable institutions and intellectual impairment c.1066–1600. *Journal on Developmental Disabilities, 8*, 19–29. Retrieved from http://www.oadd.org/Published_Issues_142.html

Stainton, T., & Besser, H. (1998). The positive impact of children with an intellectual disability on the family. *Journal of Intellectual and Developmental Disability, 23*, 57–70. doi:10.1080/13668259800033581

Stebbing, C., Wong, I. C. K., Kaushal, R., & Jaffe, A. (2007). The role of communication in paediatric drug safety. *Archives of Disease in Childhood, 92*, 440–445. doi:10.1136/adc.2006.112987

Stein, L. I., Foran, A. C., & Cermak, S. (2011). Occupational patterns of parents of children with autism spectrum disorder: Revisiting Matuska and Christiansen's model of lifestyle balance. *Journal of Occupational Science, 18*, 115–130. doi:10. 1080/14427591.2011.575762

Steiner, A. M. (2011). A strength-based approach to parent education for children with autism. *Journal of Positive Behavior Interventions, 13*, 178–190. doi:10.1177/1098300710384134

Steiner, A. M., Koegel, L. K., Koegel, R. L., & Ence, W. A. (2012). Issues and theoretical constructs regarding parent education for autism spectrum disorders. *Journal of Autism and Developmental Disorders, 42*, 1218–1227. doi:10.1007/s10803-011-1194-0

Stepansky, M. A., Roache, C. R., Holmbeck, G. N., & Schultz, K. (2010). Medical adherence in young adolescents with spina bifida: Longitudinal associations with family functioning. *Journal of Pediatric Psychology, 35*, 167–176. doi:10.1093/jpepsy/jsp054

Sterling, A., Barnum, L., Skinner, D., Warren, S. F., & Fleming, K. (2012). Parenting young children with and without fragile X syndrome. *American Journal on Intellectual and Developmental Disabilities, 117*, 194–206. doi:10.1352/1944-7558-117.3.194

Stirman, S. W., & Pennebaker, J. W. (2001). Word use in the poetry of suicidal and nonsuicidal poets. *Psychosomatic Medicine, 63*, 517–522. Retrieved from http://www.psychosomaticmedicine.org/content/63/4.toc

Stivers, T. (2001). Negotiating who presents the problem: Next speaker selection in pediatric encounters. *Journal of Communication, 51*, 252–282. doi:10.1111/j.1460-2466.2001.tb02880.x

Stivers, T. (2002a). Participating in decisions about treatment: Overt parent pressure for antibiotic medication in pediatric encounters. *Social Science & Medicine, 54*, 1111–1130. doi:10.1016/S0277-9536(01)00085-5

Stivers, T. (2002b). Presenting the problem in pediatric encounters: "Symptoms only" versus "candidate diagnosis" presentations. *Health Communication, 14*, 299–338. doi:10.1207/S15327027HC1403_2

Stivers, T. (2005). Non-antibiotic treatment recommendations: Delivery formats and implications for parent resistance. *Social Science & Medicine, 60*, 949–964. doi:10.1016/j.socscimed.2004.06.040

Stochholm, K., Juul, S., Juel, K., Naeraa, R. W., & Gravholt, C. H. (2006). Prevalence, incidence, diagnostic delay, and mortality in Turner syndrome. *The Journal of Clinical Endocrinology and Metabolism, 91,* 3897–3902. doi:10.1210/jc.2006-0558

Stoneman, Z. (2007a). Disability research methodology: Current issues and future challenges. In S. L. Odom, R. H. Horner, M. E. Snell, & J. Blacher (Eds.), *Handbook of developmental disabilities* (pp. 35–54). New York, NY: Guilford Press.

Stoneman, Z. (2007b). Examining the Down syndrome advantage: Mothers and fathers of young children with disabilities. *Journal of Intellectual Disability Research, 51,* 1006–1017. doi:10.1111/j.1365-2788.2007.01012.x

Stoner, J. B., & Angell, M. E. (2006). Parent perspectives on role engagement: An investigation of parents of children with ASD and their self-reported roles with education professionals. *Focus on Autism and Other Developmental Disabilities, 21,* 177–189. doi:10.1177/10883576060210030601

Stoner, J. B., Bock, S. J., Thompson, J. R., Angell, M. E., Heyl, B. S., & Crowley, E. P. (2005). Welcome to our world: Parent perceptions of interactions between parents of young children with ASD and education professionals. *Focus on Autism and Other Developmental Disabilities, 20,* 39–51. doi:10.1177/10883576050200010401

Strickland, B., McPherson, M., Weissman, G., van Dyck, P., Huang, Z. J., & Newacheck, P. (2004). Access to the medical home: Results of the National Survey of Children with Special Health Care Needs. *Pediatrics, 113,* e996–e1004. doi:10.1542/peds.2008-2504

Strunk, J. (2010). Respite care for families of special needs children: A systematic review. *Journal of Developmental and Physical Disabilities, 22,* 615–630. doi:10.1007/s10882-010-9190-4

Summers, J. A., Hoffman, L., Marquis, J., Turnbull, A., & Poston, D. (2005). Relationships between parent satisfaction regarding partnerships with professionals and age of child. *Topics in Early Childhood Special Education, 25,* 48–58. doi:10.1177/02711214050250010501

Summers, J. A., Marquis, J., Mannan, H., Turnbull, A. P., Fleming, K., Poston, D. J., . . . Kupzyk, K. (2007). Relationship of perceived adequacy of services, family–professional partnerships, and family quality of life in early childhood service programmes. *International Journal of Disability, Development and Education, 54,* 319–338. doi:10.1080/10349120701488848

Summers, J. A., Poston, D. J., Turnbull, A. P., Marquis, J., Hoffman, L., Mannan, H., & Wang, M. (2005). Conceptualizing and measuring family quality of life. *Journal of Intellectual Disability Research, 49,* 777–783. doi:10.1111/j.1365-2788.2005.00751.x

Swanke, J., Zeman, L. D., & Doktor, J. (2009). Discontent and activism among mothers who blog while raising children with autism spectrum disorders. *Journal of the Association for Research on Mothering, 11,* 199–210. Retrieved from http://pi.library.yorku.ca/ojs/index.php/jarm/article/viewFile/22519/20999

Sweeting, H., & West, P. (2001). Being different: Correlates of the experience of teasing and bullying at age 11. *Research Papers in Education, 16*, 225–246. doi:10.1080/02671520110058679

Tates, K., Elbers, E., Meeuwesen, L., & Bensing, J. (2002). Doctor–parent–child relationships: A "pas de trois." *Patient Education and Counseling, 48*, 5–14. doi:10.1016/S0738-3991(02)00093-9

Tates, K., & Meeuwesen, L. (2000). "Let Mum have her say": Turn-taking in doctor–parent–child communication. *Patient Education and Counseling, 40*, 151–162. doi:10.1016/S0738-3991(99)00075-0

Taylor, J. L., & Seltzer, M. M. (2010). Changes in the autism behavioral phenotype in the transition to adulthood. *Journal of Autism and Developmental Disorders, 40*, 1431–1446. doi:10.1007/s10803-010-1005-z

Taylor, J. L., & Seltzer, M. M. (2011a). Changes in the mother–child relationship during the transition to adulthood for youth with autism spectrum disorders. *Journal of Autism and Developmental Disorders, 41*, 1397–1410. doi:10.1007/s10803-010-1166-9

Taylor, J. L., & Seltzer, M. M. (2011b). Employment and post-secondary educational activities for young adults with autism spectrum disorders during the transition to adulthood. *Journal of Autism and Developmental Disorders, 41*, 566–574. doi:10.1007/s10803-010-1070-3

Taylor, S. E. (1989). *Positive illusions.* New York, NY: Basic Books.

Tedeschi, R. G., & Calhoun, L. G. (1996). The posttraumatic growth inventory: Measuring the positive legacy of trauma. *Journal of Traumatic Stress, 9*, 455–471. doi:10.1002/jts.2490090305

Tedeschi, R. G., & Calhoun, L. G. (2004). Postraumatic growth: Conceptual foundations and empirical evidence. *Psychological Inquiry, 15*, 1–18. doi:10.1207/s15327965pli1501_01

Todd, S. (2007). Silenced grief: Living with the death of a child with intellectual disabilities. *Journal of Intellectual Disability Research, 51*, 637–648. doi:10.1111/j.1365-2788.2007.00949.x

Todd, S., & Jones, S. (2003). "Mum's the word!": Maternal accounts of dealings with the professional world. *Journal of Applied Research in Intellectual Disabilities, 16*, 229–244. doi:10.1046/j.1468-3148.2003.00163.x

Todd, S., & Jones, S. (2005). Looking at the future and seeing the past: The challenges of the middle years of parenting a child with intellectual disabilities. *Journal of Intellectual Disability Research, 49*, 389–404. doi:10.1111/j.1365-2788.2005.00675.x

Tonge, B., Brereton, A., Kiomall, M., Mackinnon, A., King, N., & Rinehart, N. (2006). Effects on parental mental health of an education and skills training program for parents of young children with autism: A randomized controlled trial. *Journal of the American Academy of Child & Adolescent Psychiatry, 45*, 561–569. doi:10.1097/01.chi.0000205701.48324.26

Trute, B., Benzies, K. M., Worthington, C., Reddon, J. R., & Moore, M. (2010). Accentuate the positive to mitigate the negative: Mother psychological coping resources and family adjustment in childhood disability. *Journal of Intellectual and Developmental Disability, 35,* 36–43. doi:10.3109/13668250903496328

Trute, B., & Hauch, C. (1988). Building on family strength: A study of families with positive adjustment to the birth of a developmentally disabled child. *Journal of Marital and Family Therapy, 14,* 185–193. doi:10.1111/j.1752-0606.1988. tb00734.x

Trute, B., & Hiebert-Murphy, D. (2002). Family adjustment to childhood developmental disability: A measure of parent appraisal of family impacts. *Journal of Pediatric Psychology, 27,* 271–280. doi:10.1093/jpepsy/27.3.271

Trute, B., Hiebert-Murphy, D., & Levine, K. (2007). Parent appraisal of the family impact of childhood developmental disability: Times of sadness and times of joy. *Journal of Intellectual and Developmental Disability, 32,* 1–9. doi:10.1080/13668250601146753

Trute, B., Worthington, C., & Hiebert-Murphy, D. (2008). Grandmother support for parents of children with disabilities: Gender differences in parenting stress. *Families, Systems, & Health, 26,* 135–146. doi:10.1037/1091-7527.26.2.135

Turnbull, A. P., Pereira, L., & Blue-Banning, M. J. (1999). Parents' facilitation of friendship between their children with a disability and friends without a disability. *Research and Practice for Persons with Severe Handicaps, 24,* 85–99. doi:10.2511/rpsd.24.2.85

Turnbull, A. P., & Ruef, M. (1997). Family perspectives on inclusive lifestyle issues for people with problem behavior. *Exceptional Children, 63,* 211–227. Retrieved from http://www.cec.sped.org/content/NavigationMenu/Publications2/exceptionalchildren

Turnbull, H. R., III, Wilcox, B. L., & Stowe, M. J. (2002). A brief overview of special education law with focus on autism. *Journal of Autism and Developmental Disorders, 32,* 479–493. doi:10.1023/A:1020550107880

Twenge, J. M., Baumeister, R. F., Tice, D. M., & Stucke, T. S. (2001). If you can't join them, beat them: Effects of social exclusion on aggressive behavior. *Journal of Personality and Social Psychology, 81,* 1058–1069. doi:10.1037/0022-3514.81.6.1058

Twenge, J. M., Catanese, K. R., & Baumeister, R. F. (2003). Social exclusion and the deconstructed state: Time perception, meaninglessness, lethargy, lack of emotion, and self-awareness. *Journal of Personality and Social Psychology, 85,* 409–423. doi:10.1037/0022-3514.85.3.409

Valizadeh, S., Davaji, R. B. O., & Dadkhah, A. (2009). The effectiveness of group coping skills training on reducing stress of mothers with disabled children. *Iranian Rehabilitation Journal, 7,* 9–12. Retrieved from http://rehabj.ir/browse.php?mag_id=9&slc_lang=en&sid=1

van Dyck, P. C., Kogan, M. D., McPherson, M. G., Weissman, G. R., & Newacheck, P. W. (2004). Prevalence and characteristics of children with special health care needs. *Archives of Pediatrics & Adolescent Medicine, 158*, 884–890. doi:10.1001/archpedi.158.9.884

Vermaes, I. P. R., Gerris, J. R. M., & Janssens, J. A. M. (2007). Parents' social adjustment in families of children with spina bifida: A theory-driven review. *Journal of Pediatric Psychology, 32*, 1214–1226. doi:10.1093/jpepsy/jsm054

Vilchinsky, N., Findler, L., & Werner, S. (2010). Attitudes toward people with disabilities: The perspective of attachment theory. *Rehabilitation Psychology, 55*, 298–306. doi:10.1037/a0020491

Wachtel, K., & Carter, A. S. (2008). Reaction to diagnosis and parenting styles among mothers of young children with ASDs. *Autism, 12*, 575–594. doi:10.1177/1362361308094505

Wagner, M. M., & Blackorby, J. (1996). Transition from high school to work or college: How special education students fare. *The Future of Children, 6*, 103–120. doi:10.2307/1602496

Wanamaker, C. E., & Glenwick, D. S. (1998). Stress, coping, and perceptions of child behavior in parents of preschoolers with cerebral palsy. *Rehabilitation Psychology, 43*, 297–312. doi:10.1037/0090-5550.43.4.297

Weary, G., & Edwards, J. A. (1994). Individual differences in causal uncertainty. *Journal of Personality and Social Psychology, 67*, 308–318. doi:10.1037/0022-3514.67.2.308

Weary, G., & Jacobson, J. A. (1997). Causal uncertainty beliefs and diagnostic information seeking. *Journal of Personality and Social Psychology, 73*, 839–848. doi:10.1037/0022-3514.73.4.839

Weiss, S., Goldlust, E., & Vaucher, Y. E. (2010). Improving parent satisfaction: An intervention to increase neonatal parent–provider communication. *Journal of Perinatology, 30*, 425–430. doi:10.1038/jp.2009.163

Werner, S., Edwards, M., & Baum, N. T. (2009). Family quality of life before and after out-of-home placement of a family member with an intellectual disability. *Journal of Policy and Practice in Intellectual Disabilities, 6*, 32–39. doi:10.1111/j.1741-1130.2008.00196.x

Wheaton, B. (1990). Life transitions, role histories, and mental health. *American Sociological Review, 55*, 209–223. doi:10.2307/2095627

Whitaker, S., & Read, S. (2006). The prevalence of psychiatric disorders among people with intellectual disabilities: An analysis of the literature. *Journal of Applied Research in Intellectual Disabilities, 19*, 330–345. doi:10.1111/j.1468-3148.2006.00293.x

Whitmarsh, I., Davis, A. M., Skinner, D., & Bailey, D. B., Jr. (2007). A place for genetic uncertainty: Parents valuing an unknown in the meaning of disease. *Social Science & Medicine, 65*, 1082–1093. doi:10.1016/j.socscimed.2007.04.034

Williams-Diehm, K. L., & Benz, M. R. (2008). Where are they now? Lessons from a single district follow-up study. *Journal for Vocational Special Needs Education*, *30*, 4–15. Retrieved from http://www.cew.wisc.edu/jvsne/

Witt, W. P., Gottlieb, C. A., Hampton, J., & Litzelman, K. (2009). The impact of childhood activity limitations on physical health, mental health, and work-days lost in the United States. *Academic Pediatrics*, *9*, 263–269. doi:10.1016/j.acap.2009.02.008

Witt, W. P., Riley, A. W., & Coiro, M. J. (2003). Childhood functional status, family stressors, and psychosocial adjustment among school-aged children with disabilities in the United States. *Archives of Pediatrics & Adolescent Medicine*, *157*, 687–695. doi:10.1001/archpedi.157.7.687

Wolf, L., Fisman, S., Ellison, D., & Freeman, T. (1998). Effect of sibling perception of differential parental treatment in sibling dyads with one disabled child. *Journal of the American Academy of Child & Adolescent Psychiatry*, *37*, 1317–1325. doi:10.1097/00004583-199812000-00016

Wong, F. K. D., & Poon, A. (2010). Cognitive behavioural group treatment for Chinese parents with children with developmental disabilities in Melbourne, Australia: An efficacy study. *Australian and New Zealand Journal of Psychiatry*, *44*, 742–749. doi:10.3109/00048671003769769

Wood, J. D., & Milo, E. (2001). Fathers' grief when a disabled child dies. *Death Studies*, *25*, 635–661. doi:10.1080/713769895

Woodbridge, S., Buys, L., & Miller, E. (2009). Grandparenting a child with a disability: An emotional rollercoaster. *Australasian Journal on Ageing*, *28*, 37–40. doi:10.1111/j.1741-6612.2008.00344.x

Woodbridge, S., Buys, L., & Miller, E. (2011). "My grandchild has a disability": Impact on grandparenting identity, roles, and relationships. *Journal of Aging Studies*, *25*, 355–363. doi:10.1016/j.jaging.2011.01.002

Wooffitt, R. (2005). *Conversation analysis: A comparative and critical introduction.* London, England: Sage.

Woolfson, L., & Grant, E. (2006). Authoritative parenting and parental stress in parents of pre-school and older children with developmental disabilities. *Child: Care, Health and Development*, *32*, 177–184. doi:10.1111/j.1365-2214.2006.00603.x

Wortman, C. B., & Silver, R. C. (1989). The myths of coping with loss. *Journal of Consulting and Clinical Psychology*, *57*, 349–357. doi:10.1037/0022-006X.57.3.349

Wortman, C. B., & Silver, R. C. (2001). The myths of coping with loss revisited. In M. S. Stroebe, R. O. Hansson, W. Stroebe, & H. Schut (Eds.), *Handbook of bereavement research: Consequences, coping, and care* (pp. 405–429). Washington, DC: American Psychological Association. doi:10.1037/10436-017

Yang, Q., Rasmussen, S. A., & Friedman, J. M. (2002). Mortality associated with Down's syndrome in the USA from 1983 to 1997: A population-based study. *The Lancet*, *359*, 1019–1025. doi:10.1016/S0140-6736(02)08092-3

Yell, M. L., & Katsiyannis, A. (2004). Placing students with disabilities in inclusive settings: Legal guidelines and preferred practices. *Preventing School Failure, 49,* 28–35. doi:10.3200/PSFL.49.1.28-35

Yell, M. L., Rogers, D., & Rogers, E. L. (1998). The legal history of special education: What a long, strange trip it's been! *Remedial and Special Education, 19,* 219–228. doi:10.1177/074193259801900405

Young, B., Moffett, J. K., Jackson, D., & McNulty, A. (2006). Decision-making in community-based paediatric physiotherapy: A qualitative study of children, parents, and practitioners. *Health & Social Care in the Community, 14,* 116–124. doi:10.1111/j.1365-2524.2006.00599.x

Zautra, A. J., Davis, M. C., Reich, J. W., Nicassio, P., Tennen, H., Finan, P., . . . Irwin, M. R. (2008). Comparison of cognitive behavioral and mindfulness meditation interventions on adaptation to rheumatoid arthritis for patients with and without history of recurrent depression. *Journal of Consulting and Clinical Psychology, 76,* 408–421. doi:10.1037/0022-006X.76.3.408

Zenderland, L. (1998). *Measuring minds: Henry Herbert Goddard and the origins of American intelligence testing.* New York, NY: Cambridge University Press.

Zhang, D., Katsiyannis, A., & Kortering, L. J. (2007). Performance on exit exams by students with disabilities: A four-year analysis. *Career Development for Exceptional Individuals, 30,* 48–57. doi:10.1177/08857288070300010601

Zuckerman, M. (1999). Diathesis-stress models. In M. Zuckerman (Ed.), *Vulnerability to psychopathology* (pp. 3–23). Washington, DC: American Psychological Association.

Zukerman, J. M., Devine, K. A., & Holmbeck, G. N. (2011). Adolescent predictors of emerging adulthood milestones in youth with spina bifida. *Journal of Pediatric Psychology, 36,* 265–276. doi:10.1093/jpepsy/jsq075

INDEX

Depression
  in bereaved caregivers, 140
  following a death, 136, 137
  forgiveness treatments for, 158
  mindfulness interventions for,
    157–158
  and parental stress, 32–34
  positive psychology Internet study
    of, 159–160
  and resilience, 138
  in siblings of individuals with ASD,
    117–118
de St. Aubin, E., 124
Developmental delay, 6
Developmental disabilities, 4–9
  historical constructions of, 5–7
  life expectancies with, 135
  life stage issues with. See Life stage
    issues
  models of, 7–8
  parents' challenges with, 3–4
  terminology used for, 8–9
  working definition of, 4–5
Devine, K. A., 111
Devlin, L., 24
DeWall, C. N., 91
Dewey, D., 54
Diagnosis of disability
  learning of, 17
  parents' responses to. See Parental
    responses to diagnosis
  physicians' and patients' discussions
    about, 67–68
  uncertainty in, 24–25, 28–29, 132
Diagnostic and Statistical Manual of Mental Disorders (4th ed., text rev.;
    DSM-IV-TR), 20
Diamond, A., 124
Diathesis–stress model of disability,
    9–10, 112, 117
Diener, E., 123
Differential parental treatment, siblings'
    perception of, 53
Disability
  clinical psychologists' training in,
    170
  developmental. See Developmental
    disabilities
  impairment vs., 8, 93
Disability rights activism, 8

Disenfranchised grief, 143–145
Divorce rates, 52, 115–116
Dix, Dorothea, 6
Doka, K. J., 143
Doktor, J., 82
Dolev, S., 26
Doraiswamy, P. M., 157
Double ABCX model, 37
Double transition (bereavement),
    142–143
Dowey, A., 53
Down syndrome (in general)
  adult siblings of individuals with,
    118–119
  communication between physicians
    and parents about, 68, 69
  diagnosis of, 24
  and effectiveness of social support, 55
  health care needs with, 61
  independence of adults with, 109
  parental responses to diagnosis of,
    24–25, 29
  risk of death with, 135
  well-being of siblings of adults
    with, 117
Down syndrome, children with
  educational placement of, 78–80
  parental satisfaction with schooling
    of, 85
  well-being of mothers of, 115
Down syndrome, families of children with
  grandparents' support or conflict, 57
  intervention programs for parents, 152
  narratives of parents, 129, 132, 133
  sibling relationships in, 54, 55
Down syndrome advantage, 29
Drew, A., 154
DSM-IV-TR (*Diagnostic and Statistical
    Manual of Mental Disorders*,
    4th ed., text rev.), 20
Duckworth, A. L., 157
Dunlap, G., 97
Dunn, D. S., 93
DuPaul, G. J., 32
Dweck, C. S., 34
Dyson, L. L., 32

Eakes, G. G., 34
Ecological models of disability, 10–11
Edelbrock, C., 47

Jarvis, W. B. G., 23
Javier, J. R., 64
Jevne, R. F., 40
Jobe, B. M., 33
Jobling, A., 78
Johnson, K. J., 42
Johnston, C., 32
Johnston, L., 17
Jones, S., 126
Jongmans, M., 27
Joseph, S., 38
Jotzo, M., 22
Judge, K., 117
Juel, K., 28
Jung, A. W., 84
Justice (character strength), 12
Juul, S., 28

Kagan, C., 49
Kallikaks family study, 7
Kaminsky, L., 54
Kanaya, T., 77
Kaniok, P. E., 52
Kaplan-Estrin, M., 29
Karge, B. D., 84
Kasari, C., 78
Kasper, M. A., 19
Kato, M. M., 108
Katsiyannis, A., 77, 107
Katz, R. T., 135
Katz, Shira, 57
Katz, Shlomo, 54
Kausar, S, 40
Kaushal, R., 70
Kayfitz, A. D., 41
Kearney, P. M., 31, 43
Keen, D., 66
Kelly, B., 92
Kelly, L. M., 111
Keogh, B. K., 47–48
Kersh, J., 51
Kesper, U., 157
Kessel, L., 57
Ketelaar, M., 27
Kiecolt-Glaser, J. K., 140
Kim, S. E., 62, 63
King, G., 65, 129, 149
King, G. A., 3
King, L. A., 121, 123, 129, 130, 133, 159
King, M., 26

King, M. D., 27
King, S., 65
Kirkham, M. A., 152
Kishnani, P. S., 69
Kitchin, R., 92
Klein, E., 160–161
Klein, S. D., 125
Klinefelter syndrome, 28
Knestricht, T., 59
Knott, F., 27
Knowledge (character strength), 12
Kober, R., 107
Koegel, L. K., 160–161
Koegel, R. L., 160–161
Kogan, M. D., 62, 64
Kohler, F. W., 86
Koman, L. A., 32
Koren-Karie, N., 26
Kortering, L. J., 107
Kramer, J., 119
Krauss, M. W., 49, 85, 99, 108–109, 114–115, 117, 118
Krogstad, P., 72
Kuchey, D., 59
Kumar, P., 96

Lake, J. F., 83
Lane, H., 6, 92
Lalande, K., 139
Larson, J., 137
Larson, R. J., 123
Lasky, B., 84
Lau, C., 19
Lavee, Y., 37
Lavin, C., 143
Law, M., 65
Laws, G., 85
Lawson, H., 79
Layous, K., 157
Lazarus, R. S., 36, 153
Learning of disability. *See* Initial experience
Lecavalier, L., 32
Legal protections for children, in education, 76–77
Leggett, E. L., 34
Lehman, D. R., 137
Leidy, M. S., 95
Leigh, I. W., 150
Leiter, V., 49, 85

Marlow, N., 17
Marks, S. U., 119
Marquis, J., 86
Marquis, J. G., 100
Martin, E. W., 76
Martin, R., 76
Marvin, R. S., 23
Masters, I. B., 70
Maternal roles
    and children's social competence, 95
    and well-being, 50–51
Matson, A., 119
Maynard, D. W., 68
Mayne, T. J., 139
Mazursky, H., 45
Mazzucchelli, T., 154
McAdams, D. P., 122–124, 129, 132, 138
McBride, A., 137
McCullough, M. E., 158
McDermott-Perez, L., 18, 19
McDowell, D. J., 95
McGlynn, E. A., 72
McGowan, J. E., 17
McGuire, L., 140
McHale, S. M., 53
McIntyre, L. L., 153
McLanahan, S., 45
McLean-Heywood, D., 26
McManus, J. L., 96
McNulty, A., 70
McNulty, J. K., 160
McPherson, M. G., 64
Meaning
    construction of, 129–131
    search for, 137
Medical equipment
    access to, 64
    and parent–physician communica-
        tion, 72–73
Medical homes, 63
Medical issues, 61–74
    communicating, with medical
        professionals, 66–74
    gaining access to care, 62–66
Medical model of disability, 7–8
Medical professionals
    communicating with. *See* Com-
        munication with medical
        professionals
    in NICUs, 18

tensions between parents and,
    126–127
Meeuwesen, L., 70
Mehl, M. R., 132
Melnyk, B. M., 22
Mendoza, F. S., 64
Meng, L., 26
Mental deficiency, 6
Mental health
    of parents, 85, 114
    of siblings, 117
Mental illness
    influence of, on siblings, 117
    intellectual disability vs., 6
    and siblings' present support/future
        plans, 118
    well-being of mothers of children
        with, 115
Mesosystem context, 11
Methodological issues, 12–13, 151–152
Meyer, D. J., 125
Meyer, K., 33
Meyer, K., 118
Michie, M., 130
Microsystems context, 11
Middle Ages, 5
Midlife, well-being of parents at,
    114–115
Midlarsky, E., 55
Miles, M. S., 19, 21
Miller, Elizabeth, 65
Miller, Evonne, 45, 56
Milner, P., 92
Milo, E. M., 141, 142, 143, 145–146, 147
Milshtein, S., 26, 27
Milward, L., 85
Mindfulness interventions, 157, 158
Mindfulness training, 161
Misra, S., 86
Models of developmental disabilities, 7–8
    diathesis–stress model, 9–10
    ecological models, 10–11
    stress models, 9–10
    transactional models, 10
Moffett, J. K., 70
Mohamed, S., 153
Mohay, H., 70
Moilanen, K. L., 10
Montes, G., 86
Monzo, L., 109

ABOUT THE AUTHOR

David W. Carroll, PhD, is professor emeritus at the University of Wisconsin–Superior, where he taught courses in cognitive and developmental psychology and the history of psychology, and won awards for teaching, scholarship, and service. He received a bachelor's degree in psychology and philosophy from the University of California at Davis and a master's and doctorate in experimental and developmental psychology from Michigan State University. He is the author of *Psychology of Language*, and he has published research on the linguistic analysis of written text, the teaching of psychology, and the history of psychology. He is a member of the Association for Psychological Science, and American Psycohological Association Divisions 1, 2, and 26.